WILLIAM J. ROBINSON, M.D.

WOMAN
HER SEX AND LOVE LIFE

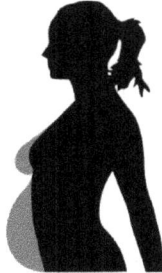

OMNIA VERITAS.

WILLIAM J. ROBINSON, M.D.

Chief of the Department of Genito-Urinary Diseases and Dermatology, Bronx Hospital Dispensary Editor of the American Journal of Urology and Sexology; Editor of The Critic and Guide; Author of Treatment of Sexual Impotence and Other Sexual Disorders in Men and Women; Treatment of Gonorrhea in Men and Women; Limitation of Offspring by the Prevention of Conception; Sex Knowledge for Girls and Women; Sexual Problems of Today; Never-Told Tales; Eugenics and Marriage, etc. Fellow of the New York Academy of Medicine, of the American Medical Editors' Association, American Medical Association, New York State Medical Society, Internationale Gesellschaft für Sexualforschung, American Genetic Association, American Association for the Advancement of Science, American Urological Association, etc., etc.

WOMAN, HER SEX AND LOVE LIFE
1917

Published by
OMNIA VERITAS LTD
*⊘*MNIA VERITAS.
www.omnia-veritas.com

© Omnia Veritas Limited - 2024

THE CREATION OF WOMAN.. **15**

PREFACE.. **17**

CHAPTER I **19**

   THE PARAMOUNT NEED OF SEX KNOWLEDGE FOR GIRLS AND WOMEN 19

CHAPTER II **24**

   THE FEMALE SEX ORGANS: THEIR ANATOMY 24

     SUBCHAPTER A.. *24*

     THE INTERNAL SEX ORGANS *24*

     SUBCHAPTER B.. *31*

     THE EXTERNAL GENITALS *31*

     SUBCHAPTER C.. *33*

     THE PELVIS.. *33*

CHAPTER III **35**

   THE PHYSIOLOGY OF THE FEMALE SEX ORGANS 35

     SUBCHAPTER A.. *35*

     FUNCTION OF THE OVARIES.. *35*

     SUBCHAPTER B.. *39*

     FUNCTION OF THE OTHER GENITAL ORGANS *39*

     SUBCHAPTER C.. *40*

     THE ORGASM *40*

     SUBCHAPTER D *41*

     THE SECONDARY SEX CHARACTERS... *41*

CHAPTER IV.. **43**

   THE SEX INSTINCT 43

CHAPTER V **45**

   PUBERTY.. 45

CHAPTER VI.. **48**

   MENSTRUATION 48

CHAPTER VII **51**

ABNORMALITIES OF MENSTRUATION 51

CHAPTER VIII **53**

THE HYGIENE OF MENSTRUATION 53

CHAPTER IX **56**

FECUNDATION OR FERTILIZATION 56

CHAPTER X **60**

PREGNANCY 60

DR. ELY'S TABLE FOR CALCULATING THE DATE OF CONFINEMENT *62*

CHAPTER XI **64**

THE DISORDERS OF PREGNANCY 64

CHAPTER XII **69**

WHEN TO ENGAGE A PHYSICIAN 69

CHAPTER XIII **71**

THE SIZE OF THE FETUS 71

CHAPTER XIV **73**

THE AFTERBIRTH (PLACENTA) AND CORD 73

CHAPTER XV **75**

LACTATION OR NURSING 75

CHAPTER XVI **79**

ABORTION AND MISCARRIAGE 79

CHAPTER XVII **81**

PRENATAL CARE 81

CHAPTER XVIII **85**

THE MENOPAUSE OR CHANGE OF LIFE 85

Change of Life in Men *88*

CHAPTER XIX **89**

THE HABIT OF MASTURBATION 89

CHAPTER XX **94**

LEUCORRHEA—THE WHITES 94

CHAPTER XXI **98**

THE VENEREAL DISEASES 98

CHAPTER XXII **100**

THE EXTENT OF VENEREAL DISEASE 100

CHAPTER XXIII **104**

GONORRHEA 104

CHAPTER XXIV **108**

VULVOVAGINITIS IN LITTLE GIRLS 108

CHAPTER XXV **111**

SYPHILIS 111

Chancroids *113*

CHAPTER XXVI **115**

THE CURABILITY OF VENEREAL DISEASE 115

CHAPTER XXVII **117**

VENEREAL PROPHYLAXIS 117

CHAPTER XXVIII **120**

ALCOHOL, SEX AND VENEREAL DISEASE 120

CHAPTER XXIX **124**

MARRIAGE AND GONORRHEA 124

CHAPTER XXX **129**

MARRIAGE AND SYPHILIS 129

CHAPTER XXXI **133**

WHO MAY AND WHO MAY NOT MARRY 133

Tuberculosis *134*

Heart Disease *136*

Cancer *136*

Exophthalmic Goiter (Basedow's Disease) *137*

Obesity *137*

Arteriosclerosis *138*

Gout *139*

Mumps *139*

Hemophilia, or Bleeders' Disease *141*

Anemia *141*

Epilepsy *141*

Hysteria *142*

Alcoholism *143*

Feeblemindedness *144*

Insanity *145*

*Neuroses—Neurasthenia—Psychasthenia—Neuropathy—
Psychopathy* *147*

Drug Addiction or Narcotism *148*

Consanguineous Marriages *149*

Homosexuality *150*

Sadism *151*

Masochism *152*

Sexual Impotence *152*

Frigidity *153*

Excessive Libido in Men *153*

Excessive Libido in Women *154*

Harelip *155*

Myopia *155*

Astigmatism *155*

Baldness *156*

Criminality *156*

Pauperism *157*

CHAPTER XXXII **159**

BIRTH CONTROL OR THE LIMITATION OF OFFSPRING 159

    Contraceptive Measures 160

    A Few Everyday Cases 161

CHAPTER XXXIII..**169**

ADVICE TO GIRLS APPROACHING THE THRESHOLD OF WOMANHOOD. 169

CHAPTER XXXIV **176**

ADVICE TO PARENTS OF UNFORTUNATE GIRLS 176

CHAPTER XXXV..**179**

SEXUAL RELATIONS DURING MENSTRUATION 179

CHAPTER XXXVI **181**

SEXUAL INTERCOURSE DURING PREGNANCY.................................... 181

CHAPTER XXXVII **183**

SEXUAL INTERCOURSE FOR PROPAGATION ONLY 183

CHAPTER XXXVIII **185**

VAGINISMUS 185

    ADHERENT CLITORIS OR PHIMOSIS 185

CHAPTER XXXIX **187**

STERILITY 187

CHAPTER XL **189**

THE HYMEN... 189

CHAPTER XLI...**191**

IS THE ORGASM NECESSARY FOR IMPREGNATION? 191

CHAPTER XLII **194**

FRIGIDITY IN WOMEN 194

CHAPTER XLIII...**196**

ADVICE TO FRIGID WOMEN, PARTICULARLY WIVES.......................... 196

CHAPTER XLIV **199**

RAPE 199

CHAPTER XLV **201**

THE SINGLE STANDARD OF SEXUAL MORALITY 201

Disastrous Effects of Wrong Teachings...................................... *203*

CHAPTER XLVI... **205**

DIFFERENCE BETWEEN MAN'S AND WOMAN'S SEX AND LOVE LIFE ... 205

Choice Between Physical and Spiritual Love............................. *207*

Love in Man Occupies Subordinate Place *207*

Polygamous Tendencies in Man.. *208*

CHAPTER XLVII **210**

MATERNAL IMPRESSIONS.. 210

CHAPTER XLVIII.. **215**

ADVICE TO THE MARRIED AND THOSE ABOUT TO BE 215

CHAPTER LXIX... **226**

A RATIONAL DIVORCE SYSTEM 226

Outsiders in Domestic Tangles.. *227*

CHAPTER L **229**

WHAT IS LOVE?... 229

CHAPTER LI... **237**

JEALOUSY AND HOW TO COMBAT IT.. 237

Causes of Jealousy *239*

CHAPTER LII **249**

REMEDIES FOR JEALOUSY 249

CHAPTER LIII... **257**

CONCLUDING WORDS.. 257

OTHER TITLES.. **259**

THE CREATION OF WOMAN

This old Oriental legend is so exquisitely charming, so superior to the Biblical narrative of the creation of woman, that it deserves to be reproduced in *Woman: Her Sex and Love Life*. There are several variants of this legend, but I reproduce it as it appeared in the first issue of THE CRITIC AND GUIDE, January, 1903.

At the beginning of time, Twashtri—the Vulcan of Hindu mythology—created the world. But when he wished to create a woman, he found that he had employed all his materials in the creation of man. There did not remain one solid element. Then Twashtri, perplexed, fell into a profound meditation from which he aroused himself and proceeded as follows:

He took the roundness of the moon, the undulations of the serpent, the entwinement of clinging plants, the trembling of the grass, the slenderness of the rose-vine and the velvet of the flower, the lightness of the leaf and the glance of the fawn, the gaiety of the sun's rays and tears of the mist, the inconstancy of the wind and the timidity of the hare, the vanity of the peacock and the softness of the down on the throat of the swallow, the hardness of the diamond, the sweet flavor of honey and the cruelty of the tiger, the warmth of fire, the chill of snow, the chatter of the jay and the cooing of the turtle dove.

He combined all these and formed a woman. Then he made a present of her to man. Eight days later the man came to Twashtri, and said: "My Lord, the creature you gave me poisons my existence. She chatters without rest, she takes all my time, she laments for nothing at all, and is always ill; take her back;" and Twashtri took the woman back.

But eight days later the man came again to the god and said: "My Lord, my life is very solitary since I returned this creature. I remember she danced before me, singing. I recall how she glanced at me from the corner of her eye, how she played with me, clung to me. Give her back to me," and Twashtri returned the woman to him. Three days only passed and Twashtri saw the man coming to him again. "My Lord," said he, "I do not understand exactly how it is, but I am sure that the woman causes me more annoyance than pleasure. I beg you to relieve me of her."

But Twashtri cried: "Go your way and do the best you can." And the man cried: "I cannot live with her!" "Neither can you live without her!" replied Twashtri.

And the man went away sorrowful, murmuring: "Woe is me, I can neither live with nor without her."

PREFACE

In the first chapter of this book I have shown, I believe convincingly, why sex knowledge is even more important for women than it is for men. I have examined carefully the books that have been written for girls and women, and I know that it is not bias, nor carping criticism, but strict honesty that forces me to say that I have not found one satisfactory girl's or woman's sex book. There are some excellent books for girls and women on general hygiene; but on sex hygiene, on the general manifestations of the sex instinct, on sex ethics— none. I have attempted to write such a book. Whether I have succeeded—fully, partially or not at all—is not for me to say, though I have my suspicions. But this I know: in writing this book I have been strictly honest with myself, from first page to last. Whether everything I have written is the truth, I do not know. But at least I believe that it is—or I would not have written it. And I can solemnly say that the book is free from any cant, hypocrisy, falsehood, exaggeration or compromise, nor has any attempt been made in any chapter to conciliate the stupid, the ignorant, the pervert, or the sexless.

As in all my other books I have used plain, honest English. Not any plainer than necessary, but plain enough to avoid obscurity and misconception.

Science and art are both necessary to human happiness. This is not the place to discuss the relative importance of the two. And, while I have no patience with art-for-art's-sake, I recognize that the scientist can not be put into a narrow channel and ordered to go into a certain definite direction. Scientific investigations which seemed aimless and useless have sometimes led to highly important results, and I would not disparage science for its own sake. It has its uses. Nevertheless I personally have no use for it. To me everything must have a direct human purpose, a definite human application. When the cup of human life is so overflowing with woe and pain and misery, it seems to me a narrow dilettanteism or downright charlatanism to devote one's self to petty or bizarre problems which can have no relation to human happiness, and to prate of self-satisfaction and self-expression. One can have all the self-expression one wants while doing useful work.

And working for humanity does not exclude a healthy hedonism; not the narrow Cyrenaic, but an enlightened altruistic hedonism. And in writing this book I have kept the human problem constantly before my eyes. It was not my ambition merely to impart interesting facts: my concern was the practical application of these facts, their relation to human happiness.

If this book should be instrumental, as I confidently trust it will, in destroying some medieval superstitions, in dissipating some hampering and cramping errors, in instilling some hope in the hearts of the hopeless, in bringing a little joy into the homes of the joyless, in increasing in however slight a degree the sum total of human happiness, its mission shall have been gloriously fulfilled.

For this is the mission of the book: to increase the sum total of human happiness.

W.J.R.

12 Mount Morris Park W.,
New York City.
Jan. 1, 1917.

CHAPTER I

THE PARAMOUNT NEED OF SEX KNOWLEDGE FOR GIRLS AND WOMEN

Why Sex Knowledge is of Paramount Importance to Girls and Women—Reasons Why a Misstep in a Girl Has More Serious Consequences than a Misstep in a Boy—The Place Love Occupies in Woman's Life—Woman's Physical Disabilities.

All are agreed—I mean all who are capable of thinking and have given the subject some thought—that for the welfare of the race and for his own physical and mental welfare it is important that the boy be given some sex instruction. All are not agreed as to the character of the instruction, its extent, the age at which it should be begun and as to who the teacher should be—the father, the family physician, the school teacher or a specially prepared book—but as to the necessity of sex knowledge for the boy there is now substantial agreement—among the conservatives as well as among the radicals.

No such agreement exists concerning sex knowledge for the girl. Many still are the men and women—and not among the conservatives only—who are strongly opposed to girls receiving any instruction in sex matters. Some say that such instruction—except a few hygienic rules about menstruation—is unnecessary, because the sex instinct awakens in girls comparatively late, and it is time enough for them to learn about such matters after they are married. Others fear that sex knowledge would destroy the mystery and romance of sex, and would rob our maidens of their greatest charms—modesty and innocence. Still others fear that sex instruction would tend to awaken the sex instinct in our girls prematurely; would direct their thoughts to matters about which they would not think otherwise; and they argue that the warnings about venereal disease, prostitution, etc., which are an integral part of sex instruction, tend to create a cynical, inimical attitude towards the male sex, which may even result in hypochondriac ideas and antagonism to marriage.

I do not deny that there is a grain of truth in all the above objections. Sex instruction does cause *some* girls to think of sex matters earlier than they otherwise would, and some girls have been made bitter and hypochondriac, and disgusted with the male sex. But it would not be difficult to demonstrate that it was not sex instruction *per se* that was responsible for these deplorable results; it was the *wrong* kind of instruction that was to blame—it was the wrong emphasis, the lurid exaggerations that caused the mischief, and not the truth. In other words, it is not sex information, it is sex misinformation, that is pernicious. And, of course, to this everybody will agree: rather than false information, better no information at all.

But if the information to be imparted be sane, honest and truthful, without exaggerating the evils and without laying undue emphasis on the dark shadows of our sex life, then the results can be only beneficent. And the task I have put before myself in this book is to give our girls and women sane, square and honest information about their sex organs and sex nature, information absolutely free from luridness, on the one hand, and maudlin sentimentality, on the other. The female sex is in need of such information, much more so than is the male sex. Yes, if boys, as is now universally agreed, are in need of sex instruction, then girls are much more in need of it. Why? For several important reasons.

The first reason why sex instruction is even more important for girls than it is for boys is because a misstep in a girl has much more disastrous consequences than it has in a boy. The disastrous results of a misstep in a boy are only physical in character; the results of the *same* misstep in a girl may be physical, moral, social and economic. To speak more plainly. If a boy, through ignorance, rashly indulges in illicit sexual relations, the worst consequence to him may be infection with a venereal disease. But he is not considered immoral, he is not despised, he is not ostracized, he does not lose his social standing in the slightest degree, and when he is cured of his venereal disease he has no difficulty in getting married. He does not even have to conceal his past sexual history from his wife. But if a girl makes a misstep the consequences to her are terrible indeed; it may not only cost her her health and social standing, she may have to pay with her very life. She runs the risk of venereal infection the same as the boy does, but in addition she runs the risk of becoming pregnant, which in our present social system is a catastrophe indeed.

To save herself from the disgrace of an illegitimate child she may have an abortion produced; the abortion may have no bad results, but it may, if performed bunglingly, leave her an invalid for life, or it may kill her outright. If she is so unfortunate as to be unable to get anybody to produce an abortion, she gives birth to an illegitimate child, which she is forced in most cases to put away in an institution of some sort where she hopes and prays it may die soon—and, in general, it does. If it does not die, she has for the rest of her life a Damocles' sword hanging over her head, and she is in constant terror lest her sin be found out. She does not permit herself to look for a mate, but if she does get married, the specter of her antematrimonial experience is constantly before her eyes. After years and years of married life, the husband may divorce her if he finds out that she had "sinned" before she knew him. And unless the husband is a broad-minded man and loves her truly and unless she made a clean breast of everything to him before marriage, her life is continuous torture. But even if the girl escaped pregnancy, the mere finding out that she had an illicit experience deprives her of social standing, or makes her a social outcast and entirely destroys or greatly minimizes her chances of ever marrying and establishing a home of her own. She must remain a lonely wanderer to the end of her days.

The enormous difference in the results of a misstep in a boy and a girl is clearly seen, and for this reason alone, if for no other, sex instruction is of more importance to the girl than it is to the boy.

But there are other important reasons, and one of them is beautifully and truthfully expressed by Byron in his two well-known lines.

> Man's love is of man's life a thing apart,
> 'Tis woman's whole existence.

Yes, love is a woman's whole life.

Some modern women might object to this. They might say that this was true of the woman of the past, who was excluded from all other avenues of human activity. The woman of the present day has other interests besides those of Love. But I claim that this is true of only a small percentage of women; and in even this small minority of women, social, scientific and artistic activities cannot take the place of love; no matter how busy and successful these women may be, they will tell you if you enjoy their confidence that they are unhappy, if their love life is unsatisfactory. Nothing, nothing can fill the void made by the lack of love. The various activities may help to cover up the void, to protect it from strange eyes, they cannot fill it. For essentially woman is made for love. Not exclusively, but essentially, and a woman who has had no love in her life has been a failure. The few exceptions that may be mentioned only emphasize the rule.

But not only psychically is a woman's love and sex life more important than a man's, physically she is also much more cognizant of her sex and much more hampered by the manifestation of her sex nature than man is. To take but one function, menstruation. From the age 13 or 14 to the age of forty-five or fifty it is a monthly reminder to woman that she is a woman, that she is a creature of sex; and, while to many women this periodically recurring function is only a source of some annoyance or discomfort, to a great number it is a cause of pain, headache, suffering, or complete disability. Man has no such phenomenon to annoy him practically his whole life.

But more important are the results of love-union, of sex relations. A man after a sexual relation is just as free as he was before. A woman, if the relation has resulted in a pregnancy, which is generally the case, unless special pains are taken it should not so result, has nine troublesome months before her, months of discomfort if not of actual suffering; she then has an extremely trying and painful ordeal, that of childbirth, and then there is another trying period, the period of lactation or of nursing and of bringing up the baby. The penalty seems almost too great.

And when the woman is on the point of ceasing to menstruate she does not do so smoothly and comfortably. She has to go through a period called the menopause, which may last one or two years and which may bring discomforts and dangers of its own. Man does not have to go through such a distinct period of demarcation separating his sexual from his non-sexual life. Altogether it cannot be denied that woman is much more a slave of her sex nature than man is of his. Yes, Nature has handicapped woman much more heavily than she has man.

In short, both in view of the fact that sexual ignorance with its possible missteps has much more disastrous consequences for the girl than it has for the boy, and in view of the fact that the sex instinct and its physical and psychic manifestations occupy a much more important part in woman's life than they do in the life of man, we consider the necessity of sex instruction much greater in the case of woman than in the case of man. I do not wish to be misunderstood as underestimating the need of sex instruction for the male—only I consider the need even greater in the case of the female.

CHAPTER II

THE FEMALE SEX ORGANS: THEIR ANATOMY

The Internal Sex Organs—The Ovaries—The Fallopian Tubes—The Uterus—The Divisions of the Uterus—Anteversion, Anteflexion, Retroversion, Retroflexion, of the Uterus—Endometritis—The Vagina—The Hymen—Imperforate Hymen—The External Genitals—The Vulva, Labia Majora, Labia Minora, the Mons Veneris, the Clitoris, the Urethra—The Breasts—The Pelvis—The Difference Between the Male and Female Pelvis.

The organs which primarily distinguish one sex from the other are the sex organs. It is by the aid of the sex organs that children are begotten and brought into the world, that the race is *reproduced* and perpetuated. It is for this reason that the sex organs are also called the Reproductive Organs.

The first thing we must do is to become familiar with the *structure* and *location* of the sex organs; in other words, we must get a fair idea of their *Anatomy*.

The female sex organs, also called the reproductive or generative organs, are divided into internal and external. The internal are the most important and consist of: the ovaries, Fallopian tubes, uterus or womb, and vagina. The external sex organs of the female are: the vulva, hymen, and clitoris. Among the external organs are also generally included the mons Veneris and the breasts or mammary glands.

SUBCHAPTER A - THE INTERNAL SEX ORGANS

The Ovaries. The ovaries are the essential organs of reproduction. For it is they that generate the eggs, or *ova*, or *ovules*, which, after becoming *fertilized* or *fecundated* by the spermatozoa of the male, develop into children. Without the ovaries of the female, the same as without the testicles of the male (to which they correspond), no children could be begotten, and the entire human race would quickly disappear from our planet. The ovaries are two in number; they are embedded in the *broad ligaments* which support the womb in the pelvis, one on each side of the womb. They are of a grayish or whitish pink color, and are about an inch and a half long, three-quarters of an inch wide, and one-third of an inch thick. They weigh from one-eighth to one-quarter of an ounce. Their surface is either smooth or rough and puckered. Think of a large blanched almond and you will have a pretty fair idea of the size and shape of an ovary.

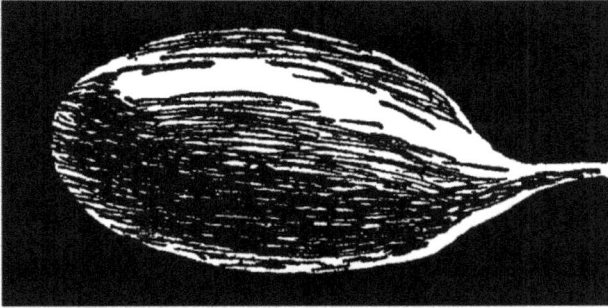

Ovary

The Fallopian Tubes. The Fallopian tubes (so called from Fallopius, a great anatomist, who discovered them; also called oviducts: egg conductors, because they conduct the eggs from the ovary into the uterus) are two very thin tubes, extending one from each upper angle of the womb to the ovaries; but at their ovarian end they expand into a fringed and trumpet-shaped extremity. The fringes are referred to as *fimbria*. They are about five inches long and only about one-sixteenth of an inch in diameter; the function of the tubes is to catch the ova as they burst forth from the ovaries and to convey them to the uterus. Taking into consideration the very narrow *lumen*, or *caliber*, of the Fallopian tubes, it is easy to understand why even a very slight inflammation is apt to clog them up, to seal their mouths or openings, thus rendering the woman *sterile*, or incapable of having children. For, if the Fallopian tubes are "clogged" up, the eggs, or ova, have no way of reaching the uterus.

The Greek name for the Fallopian tube is salpinx (salpinx in Greek means tube). An inflammation of the Fallopian tube is therefore called salpingitis. (A salpingitis has the same effect in causing sterility in the female as has an epididymitis in the male.) Salpingectomy is the cutting away of the whole or of a piece of the Fallopian tube (corresponds to vasectomy in the male).

1. Openings into the Fallopian Tubes. 2. Mouth of the Womb.

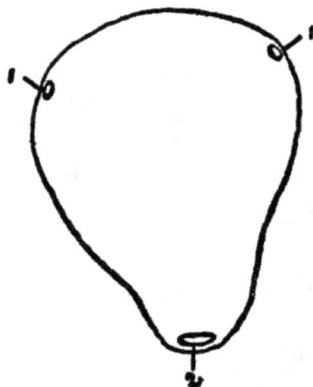

The Uterus. The uterus or womb is the organ in which the fertilized ovum, or egg, grows and develops into a child. It is a hollow muscular organ, about the size of a pear, with thick walls, capable under the influence of pregnancy of great expansion and growth. The broad part of the pear is called the *body* of the uterus; the lower narrow part is called the *neck* of the uterus, or *cervix*. The uterus in the adult girl or woman is about three inches long, two inches broad in its upper part and nearly an inch thick. It weighs from an ounce to an ounce and a half. When the uterus is in a pregnant condition, it increases enormously, both in size and in weight, as we will see in a future chapter. The cavity of the uterus is somewhat triangular in shape; at each upper angle is the small opening communicating with the Fallopian tube; the upper portion of the uterus is called the fundus; the external opening of the womb, situated in the center of the cervix, is called the mouth of the womb, or the *os*, or external os.

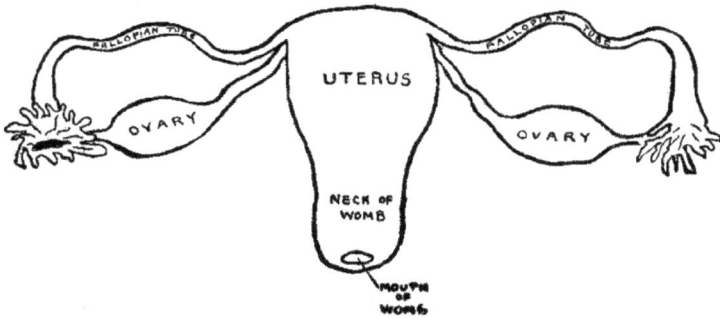

The uterus is situated in the center of the pelvis, between the bladder and the rectum. It is supported by certain ligaments, the chief of which are the broad ligaments; but, on account of general weakness, too hard physical labor, or lifting heavy weights, the ligaments may stretch, and the uterus may sink down low in the vagina, and we then have the condition known as prolapse of the womb. Or, the womb may turn forward, when we have a condition of *anteversion*. If the womb is *bent* (or *flexed*) forward on itself the condition is called *anteflexion*. If the womb is turned backwards, the condition is called *retroversion*; if it is bent or flexed backward upon itself the condition is called *retroflexion*. An extreme degree of anteversion or anteflexion, or retroversion or retroflexion, may interfere with impregnation, as the spermatozoa may find it difficult or impossible to reach the opening of the womb—the external os.

The entire cavity of the uterus is lined by a mucous membrane;[1] this mucous membrane is called the endometrium (endo—within; metra—uterus). An inflammation of the endometrium is called *endometritis*. It is the endometrium that is principally concerned in menstruation—that is, it is from it that the monthly discharge of blood comes.

The Vagina [vagina in Latin—a sheath. The vagina is the tube or canal which serves as a passage-way between the uterus and the outside of the body. It extends from the external genitals or vulva to

---

[1] Mucous membrane—briefly a membrane which secretes mucus or some other fluid.

the neck of the womb, embracing the latter for some distance. It is a strong, fibromuscular canal, lined with mucous membrane. It is not smooth inside, but arranged in folds, or *rugæ*, so that when necessary, as during childbirth, it can stretch enormously and permit the passage of a child's head. The length of the vaginal canal is between three and five inches, but it is in general much more capacious in women that have borne one or more children than in those who have not borne any.

Near the vaginal entrance are situated two small glands; they are about the size of a pea, and secrete mucus. They are called Bartholin's glands; occasionally they become inflamed and give a good deal of trouble.

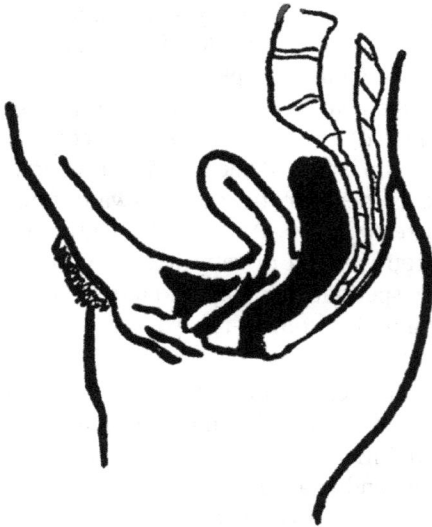

Anteversion of the Uterus.

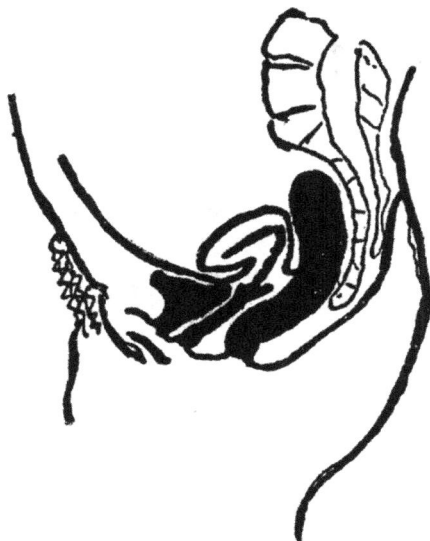

Anteflexion of the Uterus.

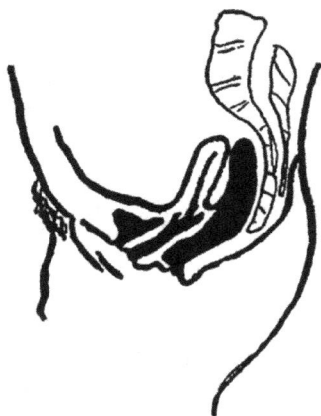

Retroversion of the Uterus.

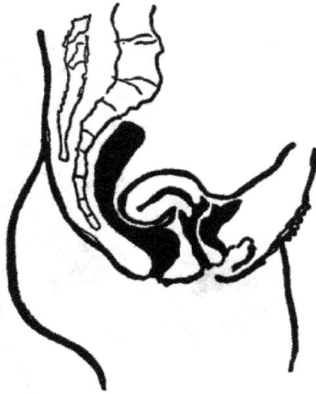

Retroflexion of the Uterus.

The Hymen [hymen in Greek—a membrane. The external opening of the vagina, in virgins, that is, in girls or women who have not had sexual intercourse, is almost entirely closed by a membrane called the hymen. The vulgar name for hymen is "maidenhead." The hymen may be of various shapes, and of different consistency. In some girls it is a very thin membrane, which tears very readily; in others it is quite tough. On the upper margin or in the center of the hymen there is an opening which permits any secretion from the vagina and the blood from the uterus to come through. In rare cases there is no opening in the hymen, that is, the vagina is entirely closed. Such a hymen is called *imperforate* (not perforated). When the girl begins to menstruate, the blood cannot come out and it accumulates in the vagina. In such cases the hymen must be opened or slit by a doctor. In some cases the hymen is congenitally absent; that is, the girl is born without any hymen. While the hymen is usually ruptured during the first intercourse, it, in some cases, being elastic and stretchable, persists untorn after sexual intercourse. It will therefore be seen that just as the presence of the hymen is no absolute proof of virginity, so is the absence of the hymen no absolute proof that the girl has had sexual relations, She might have been born without any hymen, or it might have been ruptured by vaginal examination, by a vaginal douche, by scratching to relieve itching, or by some accident.

The remains of the hymen after it is ruptured shrink and form little elevations which can be easily felt; they are known as caruncles. [In Latin, *carunculæ myrtiformes*, which means in English myrtleberry-shaped caruncles; caruncle is a small fleshy elevation; derived from *caro*, which in Latin means flesh.

SUBCHAPTER B - THE EXTERNAL GENITALS

The Vulva. The external genitals of the female are called the *vulva*. The vulva consists of the labia majora (meaning the larger lips), which are on the outside and which in the grown-up girl are covered with hair, and the labia minora (the smaller lips), which are on the inside and which are usually only seen when the labia majora are taken apart.

[Vulva in Latin means folding-door. The ancients Were fond of giving fancy names to things.

The Mons Veneris. The elevation above the vulva, which during puberty becomes covered with hair, is called by the fanciful name, *mons Veneris*, or Venus' mountain. It is usually well padded with fatty tissue.

The Clitoris. The clitoris is a small body about an inch in length, situated beneath the mons Veneris and partly or entirely covered by the upper borders of the labia minora.

The Urethra. Between the clitoris above and the opening of the vagina below is situated the opening of the *urethra*, or the urinary meatus, through which the urine passes. Many women are so ignorant, or, let us say innocent, that they think the urine passes out through the vagina. This is not so. The vagina has nothing to do with the process of urination.

Again enumerating the female sex organs, but in the reverse order, from before backward, or from out inward, we have: The mons Veneris and the labia majora, or the external lips of the vulva; these are the plainly visible parts of the female genital organs. When the labia majora are taken apart we see the labia minora; when the labia majora and minora are taken apart we can see or feel the clitoris and the hymen, or the remains of the hymen. We then have the vagina, a large, stretchable musculo-membranous canal, in the upper portion of which the neck of the womb, or the cervix, can be seen (when a speculum is used), or felt by the finger. Only the cervix, or neck of the womb, can be seen, but the rest of the womb, the broader portion, can be easily felt and examined by one hand in the vagina and the other hand over the abdomen. Continuous with the uterus are the Fallopian tubes, and below the trumpet-shaped ends of the Fallopian tubes are the ovaries, embedded in the broad ligaments, one on each side.

The Breasts. The breasts, also called mammary glands, or mammæ [mamma in Latin, breast, may be considered as accessory organs of reproduction. They are of no importance in the male, in whom they are usually rudimentary, but they are of great importance in the female. They manufacture milk, which is necessary for the proper nutrition of the infant, and they add a great deal to the beauty and attractiveness of the woman. They are thus a help to the woman in getting a mate or a husband. The projecting elevation of the breast, which the child takes in his mouth when nursing, is called the nipple; the darker colored area surrounding the nipple is called the areola.

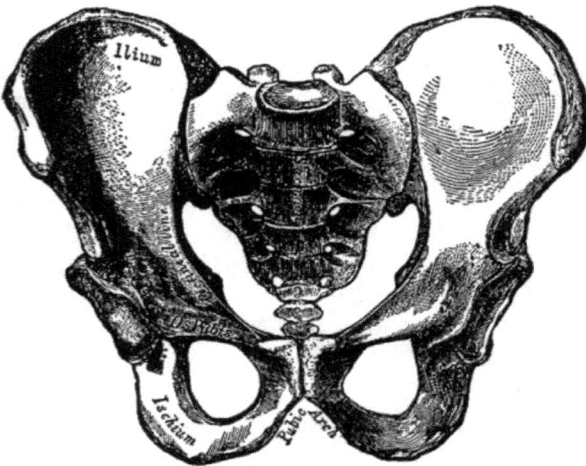

The Pelvis of the Male.

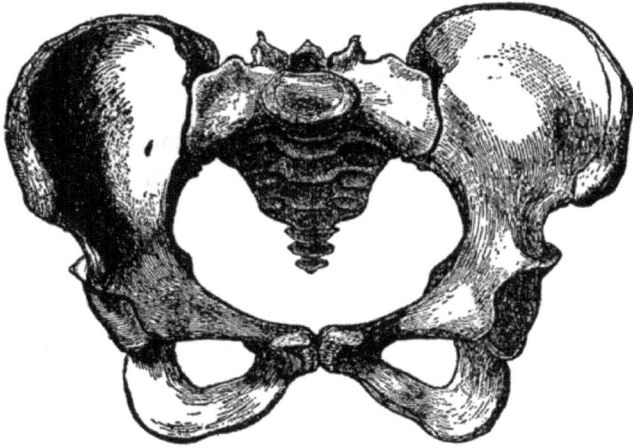

The Pelvis of the Female.

SUBCHAPTER C - THE PELVIS

The internal sex organs are situated in the lower part of the abdominal cavity, the part that is called the *pelvis*, or pelvic cavity. The meaning of the word pelvis in Latin is basin. The pelvis, also referred to as the pelvic girdle or pelvic arch, forms a bony basin, and is composed of three powerful bones: the sacrum, consisting of five vertebræ fused together and constituting the solid part of the spine, or vertebral column, in the back, and the two hipbones, one on each side. The two hipbones meet in front, forming the *pubic arch*.

The hipbones are called in Latin the ossa innominata (nameless bones) and each hipbone is composed of three bones: the ilium, the ischium, and the os pubis. The thighs are attached to the hipbones, and to the hipbones are also attached the large *gluteal* muscles, which form the buttocks, or the "seat."

The pelvis of the female differs considerably from the pelvis of the male. The female pelvis is shallower and wider, less massive, the margins of the bones are more widely separated, thus giving greater prominence to the hips; the sacrum is shorter and less curved, and the pubic arch is wider and more rounded. All this is necessary in order to permit the child's head to pass through. If the female pelvis were exactly like the male pelvis, a full-term living child could never pass through it. The two illustrations show the differences between the male and female pelvis very clearly.

Note particularly the differences in the pubic arches: in the male pelvis it is really more of an angle than an arch. Also note how much longer and more solid the sacrum (with its attached bone, called the coccyx[2]) is in the male pelvis. The differences in the pelves (the plural of pelvis is pelves) of the male and female become fully marked at puberty, but they are present as early as the fourth month of intra-uterine life.

---

[2] The coccyx consists of three rudimentary vertebræ; it is the vestige of an organ which we once possessed in common with many other animals, namely—a tail.

CHAPTER III

THE PHYSIOLOGY OF THE FEMALE SEX ORGANS

Function of the Ovaries—Internal Secretion of the Ovaries—Function of the Internal Secretion—Number of Ova in the Ovaries—The Graafian Follicles—Ovulation—Corpora Lutea—Function of the Fallopian Tubes—Function of the Vagina—Functions of the Vulva, Clitoris and Mons Veneris—Function of the Breasts—Besides Secreting Milk Breast Has Sexual Function—The Orgasm—Pollutions in Women—Secondary Sex Characters—Differences Between Woman and Man.

The importance of an organ depends upon its *function*, upon what it does, and not so much upon what it is. It is important to know the size, structure and location of an organ, but it is still more important to know its function; in other words, for our purpose it is more important to know the *physiology* than the anatomy of the sex organs.

SUBCHAPTER A - FUNCTION OF THE OVARIES

Like the testicles in man, so the ovaries in woman are the essential sexual organs. They are the fundamental organs, without which the other sexual organs are useless. Also like the testicles in man, the ovaries have two distinct functions, manufacturing two distinct substances. One function is to manufacture eggs; this, called the oögenetic or egg-producing function, is its *racial* function; without it the race could not perpetuate itself. But the ovary has also an *individual* function. Besides the ova, the ovary manufactures what we call an *internal* secretion which is absorbed by the blood, and which is of the greatest importance to the woman herself. While the manufacture of ova begins only at puberty, with menstruation, and closes at the menopause, the manufacture of the internal secretion lasts throughout the woman's entire life. This secretion, which consists of various chemical substances, has a tremendous influence not only on the development of the woman's body, but also on her feelings.

First of all it is necessary for the development of the woman's special characteristics, or *secondary sexual characters*. Without that internal secretion of the ovaries, a woman would look more or less like a man; she would not develop her beautiful rounded form, her pretty long hair, her breasts, her broad pelvis, her feminine voice, etc. *Second,* the secretion is necessary to the proper development of her other sexual organs; if the ovaries are cut out, then the uterus and the vagina and even the vulva shrivel up. *Third,* it is that internal secretion that excites in woman sexual desire and makes her enjoy relations with the male sex. If the ovaries are cut away, particularly if it is done early in life, the woman has no sexual desire and no enjoyment. *Fourth,* it contributes to the general health, wellbeing, energy, and mental alertness of the woman.

You see the importance of the internal ovarian secretion, and you will readily understand why, when the ovaries are removed by operation, the woman, particularly if she is young, undergoes such marked changes. It is because we recognize now the great importance of the ovaries that we always, when operating on diseased ovaries leave at least a small piece of ovary, if at all possible.

Number of Ova. When the female infant is born, her ovaries contain as many ova or eggs as they ever will contain. In fact, they contain more than they will at puberty. For it is estimated that at birth each ovary contains about 100,000 ova; the majority of these, however, disappear so that at the age of puberty each ovary contains only about 30,000 ova. As only one ovum ripens each month from the time of puberty to the time of the menopause (i.e., about 300 to 400 ova at the utmost during a lifetime), and as only a dozen or two ova would be necessary for the propagation of the race, it seems a superabundance of ova, an unnecessary lavishness. But nature *is* lavish where the propagation of the species is concerned. A portion of an ovary or of both ovaries might become diseased, and thousands of ova might become unfit for fertilization; nature therefore puts in an extra reserve supply. We see a still more striking example of this extreme extravagant lavishness in man; only one spermatozoön is necessary to impregnate the ovum, and only one spermatozoön can penetrate the ovum; nevertheless each normal ejaculation of semen contains between a quarter and half a million spermatozoa.

The Graafian Follicles. Each primitive or primordial ovum[3] is imbedded in a little vesicle or follicle, which is generally known as *Graafian follicle,* and there are as many Graafian follicles as there are ova. (The Graafian follicles were first described about 250 years ago—in 1672—by a Delft physician named De Graaf, hence the name.) Until puberty, that is the commencement of menstruation, the Graafian follicles with the oöcytes or primitive ova are in a more or less dormant condition. But with the onset of puberty there commences a period of intense activity in the ovaries. This period of activity is repeated regularly once a month, and it constitutes the process of *ovulation* and *menstruation.* The two processes are closely though not causally connected. Ovulation consists in the monthly maturation and extrusion of a ripe ovum; menstruation, which will be further discussed in a separate chapter, consists in the monthly discharge of blood, mixed with mucus from the inside lining of the uterus. Every twenty-eight days, from the time of puberty to the time of the menopause, a Graafian follicle bursts and an ovum is extruded from the ovary. Before the follicle bursts, it swells and enlarges and reaches the surface of the ovary; the whole follicle is congested with blood, but at one point near the surface of the ovary it is pale and thin, and here the rupture takes place.

---

[3] The ovum is really the fully mature egg ready for fecundation; before maturity it should not be called ovum but oöcyte; and in advanced treatises it is so referred to. But here ovum will do for both the unripe and ripe egg.

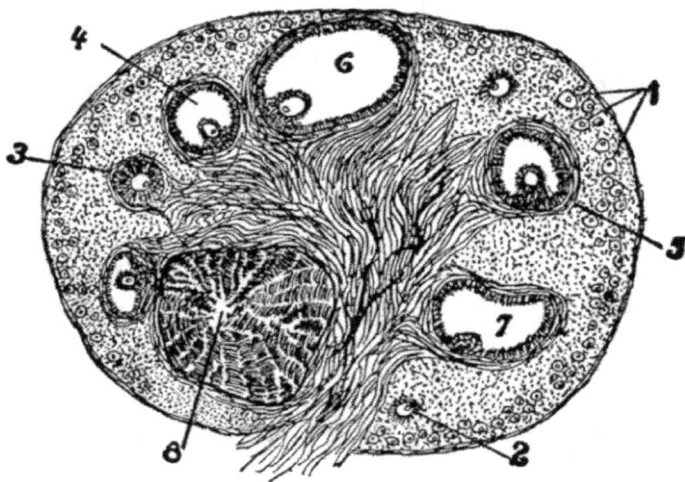

SECTION OF OVARY.
1. Graafian follicle in the earliest stage.
2, 3, 4. Follicles in more advanced stages.
5, 7. Almost mature follicle.
6. Follicle from which the ovum has escaped.
8. Corpus luteum.

Corpora Lutea. After the Graafian follicle has burst and the ovum has been pushed out, the cavity that is left does not remain empty and functionless; there is a further process going on there; there is a growth of cells, of a yellowish color, and the follicle becomes filled with a yellowish body, which on account of its color is called the *corpus luteum* (plural—corpora lutea; luteum in Latin—yellow, corpus—body). This corpus luteum grows in size until it sometimes occupies as much as one-third of the ovary. But there is considerable difference between the corpora lutea of non-pregnant and pregnant women. Up to the end of about a month the corpora lutea are the same, but after that the corpus luteum of the non-pregnant woman begins to get smaller, to shrink, so that at the end of two or three months it is reduced to a small scar and later cannot be noticed at all. The corpus luteum of the pregnant woman keeps on increasing until the end of the second month, remains about the same size until the end of the sixth month, and only then begins gradually to diminish. The corpus luteum of the non-pregnant woman, that is, the one following menstruation, is called false corpus luteum; the corpus luteum following pregnancy is called a true corpus luteum. The corpus luteum acts like a gland and elaborates a secretion which has an influence on the circulation in the uterus and on menstruation. It probably possesses other properties, with which we are not yet quite familiar. The corpora lutea of various animals are now prepared in powder or tablet form and used in medicine in the treatment of certain diseases of women.

SUBCHAPTER B - FUNCTION OF THE OTHER GENITAL ORGANS

Function of the Fallopian Tubes. The function of the Fallopian tubes or oviducts as they are sometimes called is to catch the ovum as it bursts through the ovary and to conduct it from the ovary into the uterus. It is while the ovum is in the narrow lumen of the tube that the spermatozoön which has travelled up from the uterus usually finds it, and it is in the tube, near its entrance to the womb, that impregnation usually takes place. After the ovum is impregnated or fecundated, it slowly moves down to the uterus, where it attaches itself and remains and grows for nine months, until it is ready to come out and start an independent life.

The uterus or womb is the house of the embryo almost from the moment of conception to the moment of birth. Within the thick warm sheltered walls of the uterus the child grows, develops, eats and breathes, until all its organs and functions have reached such a stage of perfection that it can live by itself and for itself. And this may be said to be the sole function of the uterus, or at least its sole useful function. For the other function of the uterus, menstruation, cannot be said to be a necessary or a useful function. It is a normal function because it occurs regularly in every healthy woman during her child-bearing period, but not every normal function is a necessary or useful function. Not everything that is is right or useful.

Function of the Vagina. The vagina is the canal in which sexual intercourse takes place. It receives the male organ (penis) during the sexual act, and serves as a temporary repository for the male semen. After the spermatozoa have reached the uterus, the vagina has no further function to perform.

Functions of the Vulva, Clitoris, and **Mons Veneris.** The vulva and the clitoris have no special functions to perform; but in them, in the clitoris particularly, but also in the labia minora, resides the feeling of voluptuousness, the pleasurable sensation experienced during the sexual act. Another seat of voluptuousness in the woman is located in the cervix of the uterus.

The mons Veneris has no special physiological function to perform, but it as well as the vulva serve as strong points of attraction for the male sex. While the entire female body is attractive to the male, and vice versa, there are certain zones which are especially attractive or exciting. Such zones or areas are called *erogenous zones*—the word erogenous means love-generating. The vulva and the mons Veneris are the strongest erogenous zones; other erogenous zones are the lips, the breasts, etc.

Function of the Breasts. The function of the breasts is to nurse or suckle the young on the mother's milk until they are able to live on other food. The other name for breasts is mammary gland (in Latin, mamma—breast), and all animals who suckle their young are called mammals or mammalia. Besides its milk secreting function, the breasts constitute a strong erogenous zone; they are a point of strong attraction for the male sex, many men being more attracted by well-developed breasts than by a pretty face. There is a good biological reason for this. Well developed breasts indicate that the other sexual organs are well developed and that the woman will make a satisfactory wife and satisfactory mother. Considering then the importance of the breasts in attracting a husband and their function in nursing the young, also their erogenous properties, it is perfectly proper to class them among the reproductive organs.

SUBCHAPTER C - THE ORGASM

The culmination of the act of sexual intercourse is called the orgasm. It is the moment at which the pleasurable sensation is at its highest point, the body experiences a thrill, there is a spasmodic contraction in the genital organs, and there is a secretion of fluid from the genital glands and mucous membranes. This fluid in women is not a vital fluid like the semen in man; it is merely mucus, and in some women it is very slight in amount or altogether absent. Adult women who live without sexual relations occasionally have sexual or erotic dreams; that is, they dream that they are in the company of men, playing or having relations with them. Such dreams are usually accompanied by an orgasm or an orgastic feeling, and by a discharge of mucus, the same as in sexual intercourse. Such a discharge of mucus during sleep is called an emission or pollution.

In the male sex pollutions play an important rôle (see the author's "Sex Knowledge for men"), because the semen is a vital fluid, and if it is lost too frequently the system is put under a heavy drain. In boys and men the pollutions or night losses may occur several times a week or even every night, or several times a night. When they occur with such frequency the man may become a wreck. Not so with women. First, pollutions or night dreams in women are much more rare than they are in men; and second, as just mentioned, the fluid secreted by woman during intercourse or during an erotic dream is not of a vital character, as the semen is in man; it is mucus, and the secretion of a mucous fluid, even if somewhat excessive, does not constitute a drain on the system. For this reason women can stand frequently repeated sex relations and emissions or pollutions much better than men can.

SUBCHAPTER D - THE SECONDARY SEX CHARACTERS

The sex organs constitute the primary sex characters. It is they that distinguish primarily one sex from another. But there are numerous other sex characters or sex differences which while not so important serve to differentiate the sexes, at the same time forming points of attraction between one sex and another. For instance, the beard and mustache are a distinct male characteristic and constitute one of the secondary male sex characters. The secondary sex characters are very numerous; one might say that each one of the billions of cells in the body bears the impress of the sex to which it belongs.

First, the skeleton. The entire female skeleton differs from the male skeleton; all the bones are smaller and more gracile; the pelvis, as we have seen before, is shallower and wider. Then the muscles are smaller and more rounded. The entire contour of the body is rounded rather than angular as in man. The skin is finer, softer, more delicate. The hair on the head is longer and of a finer texture, while over the body the hair is also finer and less abundant. The voice is finer, more pleasant, and of a higher pitch (soprano). The breasts are well developed, and serve an important purpose, while in men they are rudimentary. The breathing is also different; woman breathes principally with the upper part of the chest, man with the lower. The brain is smaller and its convolutions somewhat less complex in woman.

Woman differs considerably from man not only physically, as we have seen, but also mentally and emotionally. But into this phase of the subject we will not enter, except to remark that it is foolish to speak of the superiority or inferiority of one sex to another. In some respects man is greatly superior to woman, in others he is inferior; on the whole the sexes balance one another pretty well, and while the sexes are not and never will be exactly alike, we have no right to speak of the inferiority of one sex to another. We recognize that the sexes are different, but they complement one another, and the claim of the reactionary and of the woman-hater that woman is an inferior creature is just as senseless as is the claim made by some ultra-militant feminists that woman is the superior and man the inferior.

CHAPTER IV

THE SEX INSTINCT

Universality of the Sex Instinct—Not Responsible for Our Thoughts and Feelings.

The sex instinct, which runs all through nature from the lowest animal to the highest, is the inborn impulse, craving or desire which one sex has for the other: the male for the female and the female for the male. This instinct, this desire for the opposite sex, which is born with us and which manifests itself at a very early age, is not anything to be ashamed of. There is nothing disgraceful, nothing sinful in it. It is a normal, natural, healthy instinct, implanted in us by nature for various reasons, and absolutely indispensable for the perpetuation of the race. If there were anything to be ashamed of, it would be the lack of this sex instinct, for without it the race would quickly die out.

Not Responsible for Thoughts and Feelings. It is necessary to impress this point, because many girls and women, whose minds have been perverted by a vicious so-called morality, worry themselves to illness, brood and become hypochondriac because they think they have committed a grievous sin in experiencing a desire for sexual relations or for the embrace of a certain man. Altogether it is necessary to impress upon the growing girl, when the occasion presents itself, that a thought or a feeling can never be sinful. An action may be, but a thought or a feeling cannot. Why? Because we are not responsible for our thoughts and feelings; they are not under our control. Though it does not mean that when they do arise we are to give them full sway. We should attempt to combat them and drive them away, but there is nothing to be ashamed of, because for their origin we are not responsible.

Responsible for Actions. Our actions are under our control, to a certain extent at least, and if we do a bad or injurious act, we have committed a sin and are morally responsible. The *desire* for the sexual act is no more sinful than the desire for food is when one is hungry. But the performance of the act may, under certain circumstances, be as sinful as the eating of food which the hungry man obtained by robbing another fellow-being, just as poor as himself.

I am not preaching to you. But I am not an extremist nor a hypocrite. I am advocating neither asceticism nor licentiousness. One is as bad, or almost as bad, as the other.

What I am trying to do is to inculcate in your minds, if possible, a sane, well-balanced view of all things sexual.

For I believe that wrong, perverted views of the physiology and hygiene of the sex act and of sex morality, that is, the proper relationship of the sexes, are responsible for untold misery, for incalculable suffering. Both sexes suffer, but the female sex suffers more. The woman always pays more. This is due to her natural disabilities (menstruation, pregnancy, lactation), to her age-long repression, to the fact that she must be sought but never seek, and to her economic dependence.

For the above reasons, sex instruction is a matter of double importance to woman—this fact has been emphasized in the first chapter. But woman's disabilities impose upon us another duty: *because* she carries the heaviest burden, *because* she always pays more dearly than the man, it becomes incumbent upon man to treat her with special consideration, with genuine kindness and chivalry.

CHAPTER V

PUBERTY

Physical Changes in Puberty—Physical Changes in the Genital Organs and in the Rest of the Body—Psychic Changes—Puberty and Adolescence—Nubility.

Puberty is the most wonderful, the most significant period in a girl's life. Important as it is in a boy's life and development, it is still more so in a girl's. At this period there are often laid the foundations which either make or mar the girl's future life.

The meaning of the word puberty is maturity. It is the period at which the girl and the boy reach sexual maturity; in other words, the period at which the sex glands of the boy begin to generate spermatozoa, and the sex glands of the girl begin to mature and expel eggs or ova; with the girl puberty is marked by an additional phenomenon, which has no analogue in the boy, namely, menstruation.

Physical Changes. The word puberty is derived from the word *puber,* which in Latin means mature, ripe. But the word puber is itself derived from the word *pubes,* which in Latin means fine hair or down. For at this period of maturity all mammals (that is animals which have breasts and nurse their young) begin to develop a growth of hair. You know that our entire body, with the exception of the palms of the hands and the soles of the feet, is covered with innumerable hair follicles, and from our birth our entire body, with the exception named, is covered with fine hair. The hair may be too delicate to be seen, but it is there, and with a magnifying glass you can see it without any trouble. But at puberty the hair increases in thickness and in quantity, and becomes abundant in places where it was hardly noticeable before—the upper lip and face in boys, and the armpits and lower part of the abdomen in both boys and girls.

And so the first apparent physical sign of puberty in a girl is the gradual appearance of hair in the armpits, on the mons Veneris and the labia majora. But all the genital organs are undergoing rapid development; the vulva, the vagina, the uterus and the ovaries become larger, and the ovaries which up to that time were elaborating an internal secretion only, now also begin to manufacture ova; in other words, the monthly process of ovulation is begun. Synchronously with the process of ovulation, there commences the monthly function of menstruation. The breasts also increase in size, assume the characteristic contour, develop their glandular substance, and become capable of secreting milk for the use of any possible offspring. During this period of development they are often very sensitive to the touch or feel painful without being touched.

But not only the genital organs undergo growth and development—the entire body participates in the process. The growth in height is the most rapid at this period; the greatest growth takes place in the limbs—legs and arms. The pelvis becomes broader, and the chest or thorax also becomes broader and larger. The muscles become larger and rounder and finally give the girl the beautiful womanly form.

Psychic Changes. But the changes are not only physical; the changes that take place in the girl's psychic sphere during the pubertal years are also highly important. That is the period of the development of the emotions; she is overflowing with emotion; she becomes sensitive; in her relations with boys and men she becomes self-conscious. Distinct sexual desire fortunately does not make its appearance in the girl at this period, as it does in the boy, but she becomes filled with vague undefined and undefinable longings. It is the period of "crushes" when the girl is apt to bestow her overflowing emotion on a girl friend. There is nothing reprehensible in these crushes—they act as a safety valve—and only in rare cases are they apt to lead to abnormal development. This is also the period of day-dreaming and of romancing; the girl likes to read love-stories and novels in which she identifies herself with the heroine. And it makes quite some difference as to what the girl reads during this period, for literature has a strong influence on the young in the most plastic period of their lives; and it is important that older persons see to it that those in their care spend their time on books of noble ideals and high artistic value.

Girls of a highly sensitive or so-called "nervous" temperament, especially if there is "nervousness" in the family, must be particularly looked after. For it is during the years of puberty and adolescence that any neurotic traits are apt to develop and become emphasized. It is also the period when bad sexual habits (masturbation) are apt to develop, and the careful mother will devote special attention to her girls in their years of puberty, and guard them as much as possible against physical and emotional shocks.

The age of puberty in girls is by many writers considered as synonymous or synchronous with the onset of menstruation, which in this country in the majority of cases occurs between the ages of thirteen and fourteen. The year of gradual development before the onset of menstruation is by some referred to as the pre-pubertal year; and the first year after the onset of menstruation is the post-pubertal year. The period from puberty to full sexual maturity is called adolescence, and this term is applied generally to the period between thirteen and eighteen. For at eighteen the boy and the girl have reached full maturity. Mentally we acquire things as long as we live, and even physically the body gets larger for some years after eighteen. But sexually both boys and girls are fully mature at eighteen, though in order to become parents it is best, for various reasons, to wait to the ages of twenty or twenty-five.

Nubility. Nubility is the age or state when a boy or a girl is "fit" for marriage. This is a vague and unsatisfactory term. At the age of thirteen to fifteen boys and girls are physically "fit" for marriage, that is at that age a boy is capable of begetting and a girl of having children. But it does not mean that it would be advisable for them to marry at such an early age. Neither their bodies nor their minds are fully developed, and children begotten of such young parents are apt to be weaklings, both mentally and physically. The youngest age for girls to marry should be eighteen, and for boys twenty; but the youngest age for becoming parents should be twenty to twenty-two for the mother and twenty-three to twenty-five for the father.

CHAPTER VI

MENSTRUATION

Definition of Menstruation—Where Menstrual Blood Comes From—Age of Menstruation—Age of Cessation of Menstruation—Duration—Amount—Regularity and Irregularity.

The first function with which the girl will be confronted, which will impress upon her that she is a creature of sex, that she is decidedly different from the boy, is *menstruation*. And this function we will now proceed to study.

What is menstruation? Menstruation is a monthly discharge of blood. The word is derived from the Latin word mensis, which means a month; and menstruation is also frequently spoken of as *the menses*. It is also called the catamenia or catamenia-flow (Greek, kata—by, men—a month). Other terms are: the periods, courses, monthlies, turns, monthly changes, monthly sickness, sickness, flowers, to be unwell, to be regular. "Not to see anything" is a common term for having missed the menses. This flow of blood recurs in most cases with remarkable regularity once a month; not a calendar month, but once a lunar month, i.e., once every twenty-eight days. And as there are thirteen lunar months a year, a woman menstruates not twelve but thirteen times a year.

Where does the menstrual blood come from? The menstrual blood comes from the inside of the womb. Every month, for a few days prior to menstruation, the inside lining of the womb (what we call the mucous membrane or endometrium) becomes congested and its bloodvessels become distended with blood. If the woman has sexual intercourse and pregnancy happens to take place, then this extra blood is used to nourish and develop the new child; but if no pregnancy takes place, that extra blood exudes from the bloodvessels (some of the bloodvessels rupture) and is discharged from the uterus into the vagina, and from there to the outside, where it is caught on cotton, sanitary napkins or some other pad.

At what age does menstruation begin? The usual age at which menstruation begins in this country is thirteen or fourteen; in some it may occur as early as twelve, in others as late as fifteen, sixteen or even seventeen. For menstruation to begin earlier than twelve or later than seventeen is in this country a rare exception. But in cold northern climates the age of eighteen is not rare, and in the hot southern climates menstruation often starts at the ages of ten or eleven. Change of climate or of country will often have an influence on the menses. In the early years of his medical practice, the author had many Finnish girls as patients. It was a very common occurrence for them to stop menstruating for the first few months or even for the first year of their residence in this country.

At what age does menstruation cease? The age at which menstruation ceases is called the *menopause* or *climacteric*. It usually takes place at the age of forty-eight or fifty. In some cases it does not take place until the age of fifty-two, in others it takes place as early as forty-five or forty-four. In general, it may be said that the woman's menstruating period, during which she is able to have children, lasts about thirty-five years. And if no restraint be taken, and if no precautions be taken against conception, a woman could have twenty or thirty children during her childbearing period.

How many days does a woman menstruate? The usual number of days is from three to five; in some cases menstruation lasts only two days, in others as long as seven. As a rule, the greatest amount of blood passed is during the first two days.

The amount of blood. It is hard to estimate the exact amount of blood passed by a woman during her menses, but it reaches about an ounce and a half to three ounces. In some women the amount may reach as much as four or five ounces and in exceptional cases as much as eight ounces. Where it exceeds this amount, it is an abnormal condition, requiring treatment. The usual statement that a normally menstruating woman should not have to use more than three napkins during the twenty-four hours is correct.

The periodical regularity with which menstruation recurs in many women is remarkable. I know a woman who has not missed her menses in twenty years; during those twenty years the menses have started every fourth Friday, almost always at the same hour. I know another one who has her menses every fourth Wednesday, about seven in the morning. She skipped her periods during her two pregnancies, then they were irregular for a while, then they came back to Wednesday. Other women have their menses on a certain day of the month, say the first or the fifth, regardless of the number of days in the month (such cases are, however, exceptional). And in some women the menses are irregular: every three weeks, every five or six weeks, every six or seven weeks, etc. Some women never know when they may expect their menses, so irregular they are.

CHAPTER VII

ABNORMALITIES OF MENSTRUATION

Disorders of Menstruation—Menorrhagia—Metrorrhagia—Amenorrhea—Vicarious Menstruation—Dysmenorrhea of Organic and of Nervous Origin.

In many girls and women menstruation is a perfectly normal, physiological process. They suffer no discomfort whatever from it. They suffer no pains, no headache, no irritability, they have no admonition of its onset, until they feel the blood oozing or trickling out. But, unfortunately, this is true only of a small percentage. The majority of women have some unpleasant symptoms. Some have a headache for a day or two, some complain of a dragging down sensation, some are irritable, feel depressed or quarrelsome; some have no appetite, no ambition, no desire for work or company, while some girls have such severe pains and cramps that they are obliged to go to bed for a day or two and call in medical aid.

When the menstruation is very profuse, resembling more a hemorrhage than normal menstruation, it is called *menorrhagia*; if the hemorrhage from the uterus occurs out of the regular menstrual periods, it is called *metrorrhagia*. When the menses are skipped, or when they are so scanty that you can hardly notice any blood, we use the term *amenorrhea*. In a few rare cases the menstruation instead of coming normally from the uterus, comes from some other part of the body, for instance, the nose. Some women have a hemorrhage from the nose every month. In some a bloody discharge may come from the breasts. To such a substitute menstruation we apply the term *vicarious menstruation*. Such cases, however, are rare, and are mere curiosities.

Dysmenorrhea. I mentioned before that in some girls and women the menses are accompanied by pains and cramps. This affliction, which is the lot of millions of women, and from which men are entirely free, is called *dysmenorrhea*. Dysmenorrhea means painful and difficult menstruation. A slight pain or at least a feeling of discomfort is present in most cases of menstruation. But in many cases the pain is so severe, so *excruciating,* that the sufferer, girl or woman, is incapacitated for any work, and must go to bed for a day or two. In some cases the pain is so severe as to necessitate the use of morphine, and as it is a very bad thing to have to give morphine every three or four weeks, every endeavor should be made to find out the cause of the trouble and to remove it. It is a mistake, however, to think that all or even most cases of dysmenorrhea are due to some local trouble, that is, to an inflammation of the ovaries, or a displacement of the womb. Many cases of dysmenorrhea are of *nervous* origin; the cause resides in the central nervous system, and not in the genital organs themselves. It is, therefore, not advisable to undertake any local treatment, unless a competent physician has made a thorough examination and has decided that local treatment is advisable.

As to the percentage of dysmenorrhea, a recent statistical examination of 4,000 women showed that dysmenorrhea of some degree was present in over one-half, namely, 52 per cent.

CHAPTER VIII

THE HYGIENE OF MENSTRUATION

Lack of Cleanliness During Menstrual Period—Superstitious Beliefs—Hygiene of Menstruation.

The hygiene of menstruation can be expressed in two words: cleanliness and rest. Common sense would suggest these two measures, and as far as rest is concerned, many women do rest or take it easy while they are unwell. Some are forced to do it, because, if they don't, their dysmenorrhea is worse and the amount of blood they lose is considerably increased. The same cannot be said of cleanliness. Due undoubtedly to the superstitious opinions about menstruation, which came over to us from the ages-of-long-ago, menstruation is still considered a *noli-me-tangere*, and women are afraid to bathe, to douche or even to wash during the periods. And if there is any period when a woman needs a douche it is during menstruation. Any leucorrhea that a woman may be suffering from becomes aggravated around the periods; the menstrual blood of some women has a decided odor, and if no cleansing douche is taken during four or five days, some of the blood decomposes and acquires a decidedly offensive odor, which can be noticed at some distance and to which some men and women are very susceptible. There are some women who never take a vaginal douche. Some consider it a useless and unnecessary luxury; while some orthodox puritanical women consider it an ungodly procedure (forgetting that cleanliness is next to godliness) fit only for women of gay and questionable character. If these orthodox women knew what was good for them—and for their health—they would take a douche at least during menstruation, if at no other time.

Cleanliness. When the girl reaches the age of twelve or thirteen the mother should explain to her the phenomenon of menstruation and the likelihood of its making its appearance in a short time. Of course she should be told that there is nothing shameful in it, that when it makes its appearance she should at once tell her mother, who will instruct her what to do. She should be shown the use of sanitary napkins. Rags, unless recently washed and kept wrapped up and protected from dust, should not be used. Unclean rags may lead to infection. I have no doubt that many cases of leucorrhea date back their origin to unwashed rags. Every morning and every evening the girl should wash the external genitals with warm water, or plain soap and water. Married women should also take a douche once a day— the douche may consist of two quarts of water in which has been dissolved a teaspoonful of common table salt, or a tablespoonful of borax or boric acid. Such things like alum, potassium permanganate, carbolic acid, lactic acid, or tincture of iodine should only be used when there is leucorrhea present and generally only under a physician's directions. Bathing is permissible, but it is safe to use only a lukewarm bath. Cold tub baths, cold shower baths, as well as ocean and river bathing are best avoided during the period; at least during the first two days. I do not give this as an absolute rule; I know women who bathe and swim in the ocean during their menstrual periods without any injury to themselves, but they are exceptionally robust women; advice in books is for the average person, and it is always best to be on the safe side.

Rest. Rest is just as important during menstruation as cleanliness, if not more so. Some women as mentioned before feel during their menses just as well as they do at other times, and do not need any special hygiene. But these are in the minority. Most girls and women do feel somewhat below par during that period, and it is very important that they take it easy, particularly during the first two days. It is an outrage that many delicate, weak girls and women must stay on their feet all day or work on a machine when they should be at home in bed or lying down on a couch.

The womb is congested during the period, is larger and heavier than normal, and it is then that there is often laid the foundation for some future uterine disease, the well-known "womb trouble," or "female disease." It is not necessary that work be given up altogether, but there certainly should be less of it and there should be as much rest as possible. For delicate and sensitive girls it is always best to stay away from school during the first and second days. Speaking again of the average and not the exception, it is best that dancing, bicycle riding, horseback riding, rowing, and other athletic exercises be given up altogether during the menses. Automobile riding and railroad and carriage travelling prove injurious in some instances, greatly increasing the flow of blood. But these are the exceptions at the other extreme.

CHAPTER IX

FECUNDATION OR FERTILIZATION

Fecundation or Fertilization—Process of Fecundation—When the Ovum Matures—Fate of Ovum When no Intercourse Has Taken Place—Entrance of Spermatozoa as Result of Intercourse—The Spermatozoa in Search of the Ovum—Rapidity of Movements of Spermatozoa—Absorption of Spermatozoön by Ovum—Activity of Impregnated Ovum in Finding Place to Develop—Pregnancy in the Fallopian Tube and Its Dangers—Twin Pregnancy—Passivity of Ovum and Activity of Spermatozoön Foretell the Contrasting Rôles of the Man and the Woman Throughout Life.

Fecundation and fertilization are important terms to remember. They stand for the most important phenomenon in the living world. Without it there would be no plants and no animals, excepting a few very low forms of no importance, and of course no human beings.

Fecundation or fertilization is the process of union of the female germ cell with the male germ cell; speaking of animals, it is the process of union of the egg or ovum of the female with the spermatozoön of the male. When a successful union of these two cells takes place a new being is started. The process of fertilization or fecundation is also known as impregnation and conception. We say, to fertilize (chiefly, however, when speaking of plants) or to fecundate an ovum, or to impregnate a female or woman, and to conceive a child. We say the woman has become impregnated or has conceived.

The Process. The process of fecundation is briefly as follows. An ovum becomes mature, breaks through its Graafian follicle in the ovary and is set free. It is caught by the fimbriated or trumpet-shaped extremity of the Fallopian tube and, moved by the wave-like motion of the cilia[4] of the lining of the tube, it begins its travel towards the uterus. If no sexual intercourse has taken place nothing happens. The

---

[4] Hair-like appendages.

ovum dries up, or "dies," and either remains somewhere in the tube or womb or is removed from the latter with the menstruation, or mucous discharge. But if intercourse has taken place, thousands and thousands of the male germ cells or spermatozoa enter the uterus through its opening or external os, and begin to travel upward in search of the ovum. The spermatozoa are capable of independent motion, and they travel pretty fast. It is claimed that they can travel an inch in seven minutes, which is pretty fast when you take into consideration that a spermatozoön is only 1/300 of an inch long. Many of the spermatozoa, weaker than the others, perish on the way, and only a few continue the journey up through the uterus to the tube. When near the little ovum, which remains passive, their movements become more and more rapid, they seem to be attracted to it as if by a magnet, and finally one spermatozoön—just one—the one that happens to be the strongest or the nearest, makes a mad rush at it with its head, perforates it, and is completely swallowed up by it. As soon as the spermatozoön has been absorbed by the ovum, the opening through which it got in becomes tightly sealed up—a coagulation takes place near it—so that no other spermatozoa can enter the ovum. For if two or more spermatozoa got into the same ovum a monstrosity would be apt to be the result.

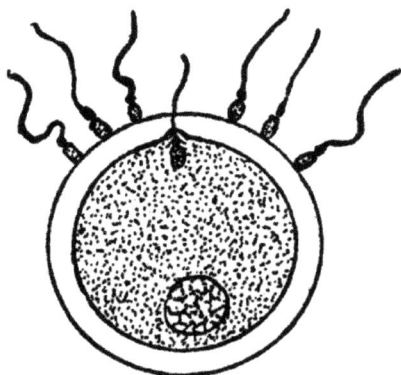

Spermatozoön Penetrating the Ovum.

What becomes of all the other spermatozoa? They perish. Only one is needed. But in the ovum that has been impregnated, and which is now called an embryo, a feverish activity commences. First of all it looks for a fixed place of abode. If the ovum happened to be in the uterus when the spermatozoön met and entered it, it remains there.

It becomes attached to some spot in the lining of the womb and there it grows and develops, until at the end of nine months it has reached its full growth, and the womb opens and it comes out into the outside world. If the ovum is in the Fallopian tube when the spermatozoön meets it, as is usually the case, it travels down to the uterus, and fixes itself there.

Extra-Uterine Pregnancy. The tube is a bad place for the ovum to grow and develop, because the tube cannot stretch to such an extent as the uterus can, nor can it furnish the embryo such good nourishment as the uterus can. Occasionally, however, it happens that the impregnated ovum remains in the tube and develops there; we then have a case of what we call *extra-uterine* (outside-of-the-uterus) or *tubal* pregnancy. Extra-uterine pregnancy is also called *ectopic* pregnancy, or ectopic gestation. Unless diagnosed early and operated upon, the woman may be in great danger, for after a few weeks or months the tube generally ruptures.

From the moment the spermatozoön has entered the ovum, a process of *division* or *segmentation* commences. The ovum, which consists of one cell, divides into two, the two into four, the four into eight, the eight into sixteen, these into thirty-two, these into sixty-four, 128, 256, 512, 1,024, until they can no longer be counted. This mulberry mass of cells arranges itself into two layers, with a cavity in between. And from these layers of cells there develop gradually all organs and tissues, until a fully formed and perfect child is the result. If two ova are impregnated at the same time by two spermatozoa, the result is twins.[5]

I might mention here that the moment the ovum is impregnated, i.e., joined by a spermatozoön, it is called technically a zygote; it is also called embryo, and this name is applied to it until the age of five or six weeks. Some use the term embryo up to two or three months. After that, until it is born, it is called fetus.

---

[5] Each ovum has one germinal vesicle; occasionally one ovum may contain two germinal vesicles; and from the impregnation of such an ovum a twin pregnancy may result.

A study of the development of the embryo and the formation of the various organs from one single cell, the ovum, vitalized or fecundated by another single cell, the spermatozoön, is the most wonderful and most fascinating of all studies. But that belongs to the domain of Embryology, which is a separate science.

What we see in the process of fecundation is a foreshadowing of the future man and woman. The ovum has no motion of its own, it is moved along by the wave-like motions of the lining cells of the Fallopian tube, and throughout the entire act it remains passive. The spermatozoön, on the other hand, is in a state of continuous activity from the moment it has been ejaculated by the male until it has reached its goal—the ovum. And as the spermatozoa carry in them the entire impress of the man, and the ova of the woman, they foretell us the fates of the future boy and girl. The woman's rôle throughout life is a passive and the man's an active one. And in choosing a mate the man will always be the active factor or pursuer. So biology seems to tell us. Whether education—using the word in its broadest sense—will effect a radical change in the relation of man and woman remains to be seen. A change putting the man and the woman on a footing of *equality* would be desirable; but whether biological differences having their roots in the remotest antiquity can be obliterated, is a question the answer of which lies in the distant future. As Geddes and Thomson so well said: The differences [between the sexes may be exaggerated or lessened, but to obliterate them it would be necessary to have all the evolution over again on a new basis. What was decided among the prehistoric Protozoa cannot be annulled by act of Parliament.

CHAPTER X

PREGNANCY

Period of Pregnancy in Human Female—Physiologic Process of Pregnancy—Growth of Embryo from Moment of Conception—Pregnant Woman Provides Nourishment for Two—Her Excreting Organs Must Work for Two.

From the moment the ovum has been fertilized or fecundated by the spermatozoön, the woman is said to be pregnant (or in French *enceinte*. This term was used very frequently and is still used by prudes, who seem to consider the word pregnant vulgar and disgraceful). Pregnancy, or the period of gestation, lasts from the moment of conception to the moment that the fetus or child is expelled from the uterus. The period of pregnancy differs very widely in different animals,[6] but in the human female it lasts nine calendar months or ten lunar months—from about 274 to 280 days. We usually count 280 days from the *first* day of the *last* menstruation. A pregnant woman generally wants to know the day of the expected confinement—for this purpose a table is appended to this chapter. If you know the first day of your last menstruation, you will see at a glance when the confinement may be expected. There may be a difference of a few days—either before or after the expected date—but for practical approximate purposes the tables serve very well.

A simple way is to count back three months and add seven days. For instance, a woman's last menstruation occurred on April 4th; counting back three months gives you January 4th; add seven days and you get January 11th, the probable date of delivery. The first day of the last menstruation was December 30th; counting back three months gives you September 30th; add seven days and you get October 6th, the probable date of delivery. The presence of a short

---

[6] For instance, in rabbits one month, in dogs two months, in sheep five months, in cows nine months, in horses eleven months.

month like February may be disregarded, as the calculation is not absolutely, but only approximately correct.

The period at which the child's movements begin to be felt by the mother is termed Quickening. It usually occurs at the middle of the pregnancy, between the 16th and 18th week.

Pregnancy is a normal physiological process; but every active physiological process is apt to be accompanied by disturbances, and there is certainly no process in the animal body in which greater activity, greater changes, go on than during the process of pregnancy. Just see what occurs in nine months. The uterus, at first the size of a small pear, reaches a size larger than that of the head of a big man; it does not merely stretch, as some think, but it actually grows enormously in size, the muscular walls of a pregnant uterus being many times thicker than those of a non-pregnant one. They have to be or they would not have the strength to expel the child, when the proper time comes. It is to be borne in mind that the child does not slip out by itself; it is the powerful muscular contractions of the uterus that push it out. If the uterus should refuse to work, if its walls were too thin or too weak, the child could not come out, but would have to be taken out with forceps. Still greater changes than in the uterus take place in the child itself. At the moment of conception it is the size of *the head of a pin*; at the moment of birth it weighs from seven to ten pounds; at the moment of conception it is a minute, undifferentiated mass of protoplasm, just a single fertilized cell; at the moment of birth it consists of millions and millions of cells, which have become differentiated into numerous harmoniously working organs, and different tissues, such as brain and nerve tissue, muscular tissue, connective tissue, bone, cartilage, etc., etc. A truly wonderful process. And in the meantime this child, which is biologically a parasite (though it is not a nice name to call it by) draws its sustenance from the mother's blood, and the mother has to provide nourishment for two. And, besides providing nourishment, her excreting organs, her kidneys, must work for two, because her system has also to get rid of the child's excretions. No wonder that the pregnant woman, particularly under an artificial unhealthy mode of living, is subject to many troubles and disturbances.

DR. ELY'S TABLE FOR CALCULATING THE DATE OF CONFINEMENT

EXPLANATION.—Find in top line the date of menstruation, the figure below will indicate the date when confinement may be expected, *i.e.*, if date of menstruation is June 1st, confinement may be expected on March 8th, or one day earlier if leap year.

	1	2	3	4	5	6	7	8	9	10	11	12	13	14	15	16	17	18	19	20	21	22	23	24	25	26	27	28	29	30	31	
January	1	2	3	4	5	6	7	8	9	10	11	12	13	14	15	16	17	18	19	20	21	22	23	24	25	26	27	28	29	30	31	NOV.
OCTOBER	8	9	10	11	12	13	14	15	16	17	18	19	20	21	22	23	24	25	26	27	28	29	30	31	1	2	3	4	5	6	7	
February	1	2	3	4	5	6	7	8	9	10	11	12	13	14	15	16	17	18	19	20	21	22	23	24	25	26	27	28				DEC.
NOVEMBER	8	9	10	11	12	13	14	15	16	17	18	19	20	21	22	23	24	25	26	27	28	29	30	1	2	3	4	5				
March	1	2	3	4	5	6	7	8	9	10	11	12	13	14	15	16	17	18	19	20	21	22	23	24	25	26	27	28	29	30	31	JAN.
DECEMBER	6	7	8	9	10	11	12	13	14	15	16	17	18	19	20	21	22	23	24	25	26	27	28	29	30	31	1	2	3	4	5	
April	1	2	3	4	5	6	7	8	9	10	11	12	13	14	15	16	17	18	19	20	21	22	23	24	25	26	27	28	29	30		FEB.
JANUARY	6	7	8	9	10	11	12	13	14	15	16	17	18	19	20	21	22	23	24	25	26	27	28	29	30	31	1	2	3	4		
May	1	2	3	4	5	6	7	8	9	10	11	12	13	14	15	16	17	18	19	20	21	22	23	24	25	26	27	28	29	30	31	MAR.
FEBRUARY	5	6	7	8	9	10	11	12	13	14	15	16	17	18	19	20	21	22	23	24	25	26	27	28	1	2	3	4	5	6	7	
June	1	2	3	4	5	6	7	8	9	10	11	12	13	14	15	16	17	18	19	20	21	22	23	24	25	26	27	28	29	30		APRIL
MARCH	8	9	10	11	12	13	14	15	16	17	18	19	20	21	22	23	24	25	26	27	28	29	30	31	1	2	3	4	5	6		
July	1	2	3	4	5	6	7	8	9	10	11	12	13	14	15	16	17	18	19	20	21	22	23	24	25	26	27	28	29	30	31	MAY
APRIL	7	8	9	10	11	12	13	14	15	16	17	18	19	20	21	22	23	24	25	26	27	28	29	30	1	2	3	4	5	6	7	
August	1	2	3	4	5	6	7	8	9	10	11	12	13	14	15	16	17	18	19	20	21	22	23	24	25	26	27	28	29	30	31	JUNE
MAY	8	9	10	11	12	13	14	15	16	17	18	19	20	21	22	23	24	25	26	27	28	29	30	31	1	2	3	4	5	6	7	
September	1	2	3	4	5	6	7	8	9	10	11	12	13	14	15	16	17	18	19	20	21	22	23	24	25	26	27	28	29	30		JULY
JUNE	8	9	10	11	12	13	14	15	16	17	18	19	20	21	22	23	24	25	26	27	28	29	30	1	2	3	4	5	6	7		
October	1	2	3	4	5	6	7	8	9	10	11	12	13	14	15	16	17	18	19	20	21	22	23	24	25	26	27	28	29	30	31	AUG.
JULY	8	9	10	11	12	13	14	15	16	17	18	19	20	21	22	23	24	25	26	27	28	29	30	31	1	2	3	4	5	6	7	8
November	1	2	3	4	5	6	7	8	9	10	11	12	13	14	15	16	17	18	19	20	21	22	23	24	25	26	27	28	29	30		SEPT.
AUGUST	8	9	10	11	12	13	14	15	16	17	18	19	20	21	22	23	24	25	26	27	28	29	30	31	1	2	3	4	5	6		
December	1	2	3	4	5	6	7	8	9	10	11	12	13	14	15	16	17	18	19	20	21	22	23	24	25	26	27	28	29	30	31	OCT.
SEPTEMBER	7	8	9	10	11	12	13	14	15	16	17	18	19	20	21	22	23	24	25	26	27	28	29	30	1	2	3	4	5	6	7	

CHAPTER XI

THE DISORDERS OF PREGNANCY

Smooth Course of Pregnancy in Some Women—Pregnancy and Parturition May be Made Normal Processes Through Education in True Hygiene—Morning Sickness and Its Treatment—Necessity for Medical Advice in Pernicious Vomiting—Anorexia—Bulimia—Aversion Towards Certain Foods—Peculiar Cravings—Tendency to Constipation Aggravated by Pregnancy—Dietary Measures in Constipation—Rectal Injections in Constipation—Laxatives—Cause of Frequent Desire to Urinate During First Two or Three and Last Months of Pregnancy—Treatment of Frequent Urination—Cause of Piles During Pregnancy and Their Treatment—Cause of Itching of External Genitals During Pregnancy and Treatment—Cause of Varicose Veins and Treatment—Liver Spots.

We saw that in some women menstruation runs a perfectly smooth course, free from any disagreeable symptoms. The same is true of pregnancy. It is remarkable how smooth and easy the entire course is with some women. Many women know that they are pregnant only because of the non-appearance of the monthly periods; and even in the later months they feel no discomfort, attending to all their work and pleasures as usual; and even childbirth is a trifling matter with them. Unfortunately the number of such women is not very large, and, because of our confined, unnatural, often exhausting way of living, is becoming smaller and smaller. There is no question that the civilized, refined woman has a harder ordeal in pregnancy and childbirth than has her primitive sister. We confidently hope that this will not be so in the future; we expect the time to come when true hygiene will be an integral part of the education and the life of every girl, and then pregnancy and parturition may become even easier processes than they are in the primitive races. But the time is not yet; and in the meantime our young women have a good deal to go through.

Morning Sickness. One of the commonest disorders of pregnancy is the so-called morning sickness. This consists in a feeling of nausea and vomiting, which comes on soon after getting up. The morning sickness makes its first appearance in the third, fourth or fifth week of pregnancy and lasts usually until the end of the third or fourth month. In some women, however, the morning sickness comes on in a few days after impregnation has taken place, and those women diagnose their condition unmistakably by the feeling of slight nausea which they experience on getting up. Medicines are as a rule of little use in treating morning sickness. The "disease" can be relieved but not cured. The patient should stay in bed later than usual, should have her breakfast in bed, and then not get up for about half an hour afterward. If the patient is anemic, a good iron preparation may prove useful.

Pernicious Vomiting. The vomiting of pregnancy sometimes becomes so severe and uncontrollable that it has been given the name pernicious. The patient is unable to retain any kind of food, not even liquids, vomits almost incessantly, and may become very much run down and exhausted. The vomited matter may contain blood. For this condition a competent physician must be consulted, for in some cases the patient's life may be in danger and an abortion has to be performed.

Capricious Appetite. A capricious appetite is very common in pregnancy. The capriciousness may express itself in four different directions: (1) The patient may lose her appetite, almost altogether, partaking only of very little food, and that with effort. This condition of loss of appetite is called anorexia. (2) The patient may develop an enormous appetite—what we call bulimia—eating several times as much as she does ordinarily. (3) She may develop an aversion towards certain articles of food. Thus many women develop an aversion towards meat, the mere sight of or talk about meat causing in them a sensation of nausea. (4) She may show a craving for the most peculiar articles of food and for articles which are not food at all. The craving for sour pickles or sour cabbage is well-known; but some women will eat chalk, sand, and even more peculiar things (for the chalk there may be a reason: the system needs an extra amount of lime and chalk is carbonate of lime).

Constipation. Constipation is very common among women in the non-pregnant condition; but in the pregnant it is much more common and much more aggravated. Constipation must be guarded against, but the measures must be of a mild nature. If we can relieve the constipation by dietary measures alone, so much the better. The dietary measures should consist in eating plenty of fruit—prunes, apples, figs, dates, etc., and coarse bread and bran. Constipating articles, such as cheese or coffee, should be eliminated. Where dietary measures alone are insufficient, the patient should take an enema—a rectal injection—twice or three times a week. The enema should consist of about 8 ounces (half a pint) of cold or lukewarm water containing a pinch of salt, and should be retained about ten minutes. Instead of water, we may advise an occasional enema of two to four drams of glycerin. Or instead of a glycerin enema, a glycerin suppository may be used. If internal laxatives are to be used, only the mildest and non-griping preparations should be employed The best are: a good mineral oil—one or two tablespoonfuls on going to bed, or fluid extract of cascara sagrada, one-half to one teaspoonful on going to bed. It is very important, whatever we use, *not* to use the same thing for a long time. If the same drug or measure is used without any change, the bowels get used to it and cease to respond and we have to use larger and larger doses. In fighting constipation we must therefore constantly change our weapons: one night we use mineral oil, the next night cascara sagrada, the third night an enema, the fourth night a glycerin injection or suppository, the fifth night perhaps nothing at all, the sixth night a blue mass pill, the seventh morning a Seidlitz powder, then a rest for a day or two, then a repetition of the same measures. But always remember: first try to get along without any drugs at all. Many cases can get relieved of their constipation by a proper change in diet alone. And where this is impossible, then use mild laxatives and use them interchangeably.

Toothache is not uncommon in pregnancy, and a pregnant woman should have her teeth put in first-class condition.

Difficulty in Urination. Pregnant women often suffer with frequency and urgency of urination. Some have to urinate, while they are on their feet, every few minutes. This is due to the fact that during the first two or three months of pregnancy the uterus is not only enlarged but is also *anteverted,* that is *turned forward* and *presses down* upon the bladder. When the woman is lying down the pressure on the bladder is relieved, and she does not have to urinate frequently. This pressure lasts only the first two or three months, because after that the growing womb lifts itself out of the pelvis, rising into the abdominal cavity; it is no longer anteverted and the pressure on the bladder is relieved. During the last months of the pregnancy there is again frequent urination, because then the heavy uterus sinks again into the pelvic cavity and presses upon the bladder. The treatment for this frequent urination consists in wearing a well fitting abdominal belt or corset, which raises the uterus and prevents pressure on the bladder. Sometimes a pessary which prevents the anteversion is efficient. In all cases lying down and resting is useful. In short, keeping off one's feet is the most efficient remedy for the treatment of frequent urination in pregnant women.

Hemorrhoids (Piles). On account of the pressure of the womb on the rectum, and also on account of the constipation which is so frequent during pregnancy, hemorrhoids or piles are quite frequent among pregnant women. The treatment of hemorrhoids consists in removing the cause: wearing a well-fitting abdominal belt, and relieving the constipation. Injecting into the rectum about half a pint of cold water three times a day is very useful. For the intolerable itching sometimes present in hemorrhoids the following ointment will be found very grateful: menthol, 5 grains; calomel, 10 grains; bismuth subnitrate, 30 grains; resorcin, 10 grains; oil of cade, 15 grains; cold cream, one ounce. The piles (the hemorrhoids) are to be well cleansed with hot water, and this ointment is to be well smeared over; a little is pushed into the rectum, and a piece of cotton is put over the anus. This protects the clothes from soiling and keeps the medicine in place for a longer time. Instead of ointment a cocoa butter suppository may be used. A suppository of the following composition is good: powdered nutgalls, 3 grains; oil of cade, 3 drops; resorcin, 1 grain; bismuth subnitrate, 5 grains; cocoa butter, 20 grains. One such suppository to be inserted three times a day. The ointment and the suppository given above, if used in conjunction with the proper regulation of the bowels, will not only relieve but will cure most cases of hemorrhoids caused by pregnancy.

Itching of the Vulva. Pruritus Vulvæ. Itching of the external genitals during pregnancy is not uncommon. This may be due to the fact that the vulva is generally congested and swollen during pregnancy or it may be caused by an increased leucorrheal discharge. The itching is sometimes very severe, and if the patient scratches with her nails and produces bleeding, she may cause an infection of the parts. The patient should be cautioned against scratching; she should try simple measures to relieve the itching. A small towel or gauze compress wrung out of boiling water and applied to the vulva several times a day, followed by a free application of stearate of zinc powder is often efficient. If it is not, the following salve may be tried: carbolic acid, 10 grains; menthol, 5 grains; resorcin, 15 grains; zinc oxide, 1 dram; and white vaseline, one ounce. In very severe cases the vulva should be painted with a solution of silver nitrate, 25 grains to 1 ounce of distilled water.

Varicose Veins. In most women during pregnancy the veins in the legs become somewhat enlarged. This is due to the pressure of the womb, which interferes with the circulation. If the veins become very prominent, swollen and tortuous, they are called varicose. This condition should be prevented, because it often and to some degree always persists permanently even after the pregnancy is over. The best precautionary measure is for the woman to wear a well-fitting abdominal belt or maternity corset, which supports the womb and does not permit it to sink too low into the pelvis. If varicose veins have been permitted to develop, the woman should wear well-fitting rubber stockings, or at least have the legs bandaged with woven elastic bandages. The bandage must be applied by a competent person, uniformly and not too tightly. Constipation has also a bad effect in making varicose veins worse; the bowels should therefore also be looked after. In some severe cases all measures are of little value unless the patient at the same time stays in bed or on a couch for a few days, with the legs elevated.

Swelling of the feet should be at once attended to. It may be a trifling matter due only to pressure of the womb; then again it may be due to some kidney trouble. The physician will determine the true cause and prescribe the appropriate treatment.

Liver Spots. Chloasma. In some cases irregular brownish patches or splotches develop on the skin around the breasts, on the sides, or on the face. These patches are known popularly as liver spots or in medical language as *chloasma*. Nothing can be done for them, but they generally disappear after the pregnancy is over. A few patches here and there may remain permanently.

CHAPTER XII

WHEN TO ENGAGE A PHYSICIAN

Necessity for the Pregnant Woman Immediately Placing Herself Under Care of Physician and Remaining Under His Care During Entire Period.

The disorders and disturbances described above are, with the exception of pernicious vomiting, of a minor nature. They are annoying, may cause considerable discomfort and suffering, but they do not endanger the life of the woman or of the child. Occasionally, however, fortunately not very often, the kidneys become affected, and for this condition treatment by a physician is absolutely necessary. In fact, the correct and safe thing for a woman to do is to consult a physician as soon as she knows she is pregnant, and have him take care of her during the entire pregnancy. Some women engage a physician during the eighth or ninth month and this is decidedly wrong, because it may then be too late to correct certain troubles which if taken at the outset could have been easily cured; while many troubles in the hands of a competent physician can be prevented altogether. I must therefore reiterate: every woman should engage a physician from the beginning of her pregnancy, or at least during the third or fourth and certainly not later than the fifth month. He will examine the urine every month and make sure that the kidneys are in order, he will make sure that the child is in a normal position, and will prevent a host of other ills.

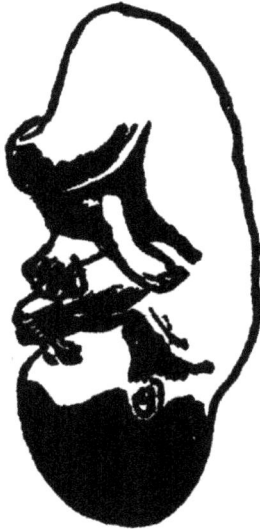

Position of the Child in the Womb.

This is not a special treatise on the management of pregnancy, and therefore minute details are out of place. Besides, to the details the physician will attend. But some hints regarding diet and general hygiene will prove useful.

If everything is satisfactory, if there is no severe vomiting, kidney trouble, etc., the usual mixed diet may continue. The only changes I would make are the following: Drink plenty of hot water during entire course of pregnancy: a glass or two in the morning, two or three glasses in the afternoon, the same at night. From six to twelve glasses may be consumed. Also plenty of milk, buttermilk and fermented milk. Plenty of fruit and vegetables. Meat only once a day. For the tendency to constipation, whole wheat bread, rye bread, bread baked of bran or bran with cream.

As to exercise, either extreme must be avoided. Some women think that as soon as they become pregnant, they must not move a muscle; they are to be put in a glass case, and kept there to the day of delivery. Other women, on the other hand, of the ultramodern type, indulge in strenuous exercise and go out on long fatiguing walks up to the last day. Either extreme is injurious. The right way is moderate exercise, and short, non-fatiguing walks.

Bathing may be kept up to the day of delivery. But warm baths, particularly during the last two or three months, are preferable to cold baths.

CHAPTER XIII

THE SIZE OF THE FETUS

Approximately Correct Measurements and Weight of Fetus at End of Each Month of Pregnancy.

Men and women are always interested to know how large the fetus is and how far it is developed during the various months of pregnancy. Absolutely exact measurements cannot be given, but the following approximate measurements are correct:

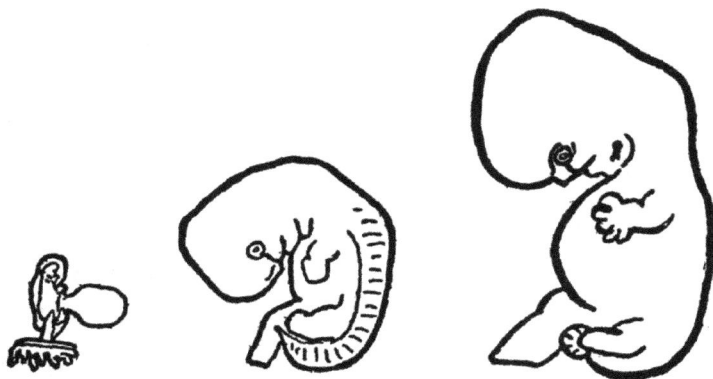

1. Embryo Between One and Two Weeks Old.
2. Embryo About Four Weeks Old.
3. Embryo About Six Weeks Old.

At the end of the first month (lunar) it is about the size of a hazelnut. Weighs about 15 grains.

At the end of the second month it is the size of a small hen's egg. The internal organs are partially formed, it begins to assume a human shape, but the sex cannot yet be differentiated. Up to the fifth or sixth week it does not differ much in appearance from the embryos of other animals.

At the end of the third month it is the size of a large goose egg; it is about two to three and a half inches long. Weighs about one ounce.

At the end of the fourth month the fetus is between six and seven inches long and weighs about five ounces.

At the end of the fifth month the fetus is between seven and eleven inches long, and weighs eight to ten ounces.

At the end of the sixth month it is eleven to thirteen inches long and weighs one and one-half to two pounds. If born, is capable of living a few minutes, and it is reported that some six months' children have been incubated.

At the end of the seventh month the fetus is from thirteen to fifteen or sixteen inches long and weighs about three pounds. Is capable of independent life, but must be brought up with great care, usually in an incubator.

At the end of the eighth month the length is from fifteen to seventeen inches, and weight from three to five pounds.

At the end of the ninth month the length of the fetus is from sixteen to seventeen and one-half inches, and weight from five to seven pounds.

At the end of the tenth lunar month (at birth) the length of the child is from seventeen to nineteen inches and the weight from six to twelve pounds; the average is seven and a quarter, but there are full term children weighing less than six pounds and more than twelve; but these are exceptions.

CHAPTER XIV

THE AFTERBIRTH (PLACENTA) AND CORD

How the Afterbirth Develops—Bag of Waters—Umbilical Cord—The Navel—Fetus Nourished by Absorption—Fetus Breathes by Aid of Placenta—No Nervous Connection Between Mother and Child.

Whatever part of the womb the ovum attaches itself to is stimulated to intense activity, to growth. Numerous bloodvessels begin to grow and that part of the lining membrane with its numerous bloodvessels constitute the placenta, or as it is commonly called *afterbirth*, because it comes out *after* the *birth* of the child. From the placenta there is also reflected a membrane over the ovum, so as to give it additional protection. That membrane forms a complete bag over the fetus; this bag becomes filled with liquid, so that the fetus floats freely in a bag of waters; this bag bursts only during childbirth. The fetus is not attached close to the placenta, but is, so to say, suspended from it by a *cord*, which is called the *umbilical cord*. When the child is born, the umbilical cord is cut, and the scar or depression in the abdomen where the umbilical cord was attached constitutes the navel or umbilicus (in slang language—button or belly button). The umbilical cord consists of two arteries and one vein embedded in a gelatin like substance and enveloped by a membrane, and it is through the umbilical cord that the blood from the placenta is brought to and carried from the fetus. The blood of the fetus and the blood of the mother do not mix; the bloodvessels are separated by thin walls, and it is through these thin walls that the fetal blood receives the ingredients it needs from the mother's blood. In other words, it receives its nourishment from the mother by *absorption* or *osmosis*. The blood from the placenta also furnishes the fetal blood with oxygen, so that the fetus breathes by the aid of the placenta, and not through its own lungs.

It is well to remember that there is absolutely no nervous connection between mother and child. There are no nerves whatever in the umbilical cord, so that the nervous systems of the fetus and of the mother are entirely distinct and separate. And this will explain why certain nervous impressions and shocks received by the mother are not readily transmitted to the child. It is only through changes in the mother's blood that the fetus can be influenced. As will be seen in a later chapter we are skeptical about "maternal impressions."

CHAPTER XV

LACTATION OR NURSING

No Perfect Substitute for Mother's Milk—When Nursing is Injurious to Mother and Child—Modified Milk—Artificial Foods—Care Essential in Selecting Wet Nurse—Suckling Child Benefits Mother—Reciprocal Affection Strengthened by Nursing—Sexual Feelings While Nursing—Alcoholics are Injurious—Attention to Condition of Nipples During Pregnancy Essential—Treatment of Sunken Nipples—Treatment of Tender Nipples—Treatment of Cracked Nipples—How to Stop the Secretion of Milk When Necessary—Menstruation While Nursing—Pregnancy in the Nursing Woman.

Every mother should nurse her child—if she can. There is no perfect substitute for mother's milk. There is only one excuse for a mother not nursing—that is when she has no milk, or when the quality of the milk is so poor that the child does not thrive on it, or when the mother is run down, is threatened with or is suffering with tuberculosis, etc. In such cases the nursing would prove injurious to both mother and child.

When the mother cannot nurse the child, it should be brought up artificially on modified cow's milk. Formulas for modified milk have been worked out for every month of the child's life, and if the formulas are carefully followed, and the bottle and nipples are properly sterilized, the child should have no trouble, but should thrive and grow like on good mother's milk. If the child is sickly or delicate and does not thrive on modified cow's milk or on the other artificial foods, such as Horlick's malted milk, or Nestlé's food, then a wet nurse may become necessary. But before engaging a wet nurse great care should be taken to make sure that she is healthy, that the age of her child is approximately the same as the age of the child which she is about to nurse, and particularly that she is free from any syphilitic taint. One, two or more Wassermann tests should be made to settle the question definitely.

Mothers should bear in mind that suckling the child is good not only for the child, but for the mother as well. Lactation helps the *involution* of the uterus: the uterus of a nursing mother returns more quickly and more perfectly to its normal ante-pregnant condition than the uterus of the mother who cannot or will not nurse her child.

It is asserted that the reciprocal affection between mother and child is greater in cases in which the child suckled its mother's breast. This is quite likely. It is also asserted that the nursing mother transmits certain traits to its child, which the non-nursing mother cannot. This is merely a hypothesis without any scientific proof.

On the other hand, the statement that many women experience decidedly pleasurable sexual feelings while nursing seems to be well substantiated.

That the mother who nurses her child should partake of sufficient nourishment goes without saying. But the advice often given to nursing mothers to partake of beer, ale or wine is a bad one. It is a question if a mother partaking of considerable quantities of alcoholic beverages may not transmit the taste for alcohol to her children. No, alcoholics should be left alone, but milk, eggs, meat, fruit and vegetables should be partaken of in abundance.

Preparing the Nipples. For the infant to be able to nurse properly the nipples of the breast must be in good condition. If the nipples are sunken, depressed, it is torture for the child to nurse. It uses up a lot of energy uselessly, becomes exhausted, and gets very little milk; while if the nipples be tender or cracked the process of nursing is a torture for the mother.

It is therefore necessary to attend to the nipples in due time—to begin at the fifth or sixth month is not too early. If the nipples are sufficiently prominent, little need be done for them except to wash them with a little boric acid solution (one teaspoonful of boric acid to a glass of water) occasionally, and now and then to rub in a little petrolatum, plain or borated. But if the nipples are sunken so that they are below the surface of the breast, or if they are only slightly above the surface of the breast, they must be treated. Gentle traction must be made on them with the fingers three or four times a day. There are only a few cases where persistent manipulation will not develop the nipple and make it stand out prominently.

If the nipple is tender it should be washed two or three times a day with a mixture of alcohol and water; one part of alcohol to three parts of water is sufficient. In washing the nipple with this diluted alcohol it should be dried and a little petrolatum or vaseline rubbed in. This done two or three times a day during the last month or two of the pregnancy will generally produce a good healthy nipple.

The Treatment of Cracked Nipples. If the care of the nipple has been neglected, and it develops cracks or fissures so that the nursing of the child causes the mother severe pain, the nursing should be done through a nipple shield, and in the meantime between the nursings the nipple should be rubbed with the following preparation, which is excellent and which I can fully recommend: thymol iodide, ½ dram; olive oil, ½ ounce. This should be applied every hour to the nipple and covered with a little cotton; before each nursing, however, it must be well washed off with warm water or warm boric acid solution. When the nipples are cracked, the infant's lips should also before nursing be carefully wiped out with boric acid solution. For the baby's mouth contains bacteria which while harmless in themselves may if they get into the cracks of the nipple set up an inflammation of the breast or "mastitis" and cause an abscess. If the cracks are excruciatingly painful, as they sometimes are, it is necessary to give the one breast a rest for twenty-four hours and have the child nurse at the other until the cracks have partially healed.

When It Is Necessary to Dry Up the Breasts. In case of the death of the child, or if the mother for some other reason finds herself unable to nurse, such as in cases where there is absolutely no nipple, instead of the prominence of the nipple there being a deep depression, it becomes necessary to stop the secretion of the milk, or as it is said in common parlance, "to dry up the breasts." In former days, not so very long ago, and the practice is still common enough to call attention to it and to condemn it, the breasts used to be tightly bandaged, or they used to be pumped every few hours. The first causes unnecessary pain and trouble, while the second procedure, the pumping, does exactly the reverse to what it is intended to do. Instead of drying up the breasts it keeps up the secretion. The best thing to do in a case like that is to leave the breasts alone, not to pump them, but just gently support them with a bandage and then in three or four days the secretion of the milk will gradually disappear.

There is some discomfort the first twenty-four or forty-eight hours, but if left alone the discomfort is less than if the breasts are manipulated, bandaged or pumped.

Menstruation or Pregnancy While Nursing. Many women do not menstruate and do not become pregnant while they are nursing. Some women will not conceive, no matter how long they may nurse the child—a year or two or longer. And some women take advantage of this fact, and in order to avoid another child they will keep up the nursing as long as possible. In Egypt and other Oriental countries where our means for the prevention of conception are unknown, it is no rare sight to see a child three or four years old interrupting his work or his play and running up to suckle his mother's breast. But not all women have this good luck. Some women (about fifty per cent.) begin to menstruate in the sixth month of lactation, while some become pregnant even before they begin to menstruate. It only too often happens that a woman considering lactation her safeguard omits to use any precautions and finds herself, to her great discomfiture, in a pregnant condition.

When a nursing woman discovers that she is pregnant she should give up nursing at once. The milk is apt to become of poor quality, but even where this is not the case, it is too much for a woman to feed one child in the uterus and one at the breast.

CHAPTER XVI

ABORTION AND MISCARRIAGE

Definition of Word Abortion—Definition of Word Miscarriage—Spontaneous Abortion—Induced Abortion—Therapeutic Abortion—Criminal Abortion—Missed Abortion—Habitual Abortion—Syphilis as Cause of Abortion and Miscarriage—Dangers of Abortion—Abortion an Evil.

The word abortion, used somewhat loosely, signifies the premature expulsion of the fetus; the expulsion of the fetus from the womb before it is viable, i.e., before it is capable of living independently. Used in a stricter sense, the word abortion is applied to the expulsion of the fetus up to the end of the 16th week; to the expulsion of the fetus between the 16th and the 28th week the term miscarriage is applied; and when the expulsion of the fetus takes place after the 28th week, but before full term, we use the term premature labor. The laity does not like the term abortion, as it is under the impression that the term always signifies criminal abortion; it therefore prefers to use the term miscarriage ("miss"), regardless of the time at which the expulsion of the fetus takes place.

When an abortion (or miscarriage) takes place by itself, without any outside aid, we call it *spontaneous abortion*. When it is brought on by artificial means, whether by the woman herself or by somebody else, we call it *induced* abortion. When an abortion is induced for the purpose of saving the woman's life, we call it *therapeutic* abortion; this is considered perfectly legal and proper. But where an abortion is induced merely to save an unmarried mother's reputation, or because the married mother is too poor or too weak to have any more children, or is reluctant to have any (or any more) for any other reason, it is called *criminal* or *illegal* abortion, and, if discovered, subjects the mother and the person who produced the abortion to severe punishment.

When the fetus for some reason dies in its mother's womb, it is generally expelled within a few hours or days. Sometimes this is not the case, and the dead fetus is retained for several weeks, or months or even years; to such a phenomenon we apply the term *missed* abortion. Some women suffer from what might be called the abortion habit; they can hardly ever carry a child to full term, but lose it in the same month or even in the same week of gestation during each pregnancy; we call this habitual abortion. And this habitual abortion may be independent of disease, such, for instance, as syphilis. The terms *threatened, imminent* and *inevitable* abortion require no further explanation.

The Causes of Abortion. Outside of the abortion habit, which may be due partly to heredity or be caused by a diseased condition of the lining membrane of the uterus, the principal cause of abortion and miscarriage is syphilis. And when a woman has had two or three or four or more miscarriages in succession we generally assume the cause to be syphilis, and in most cases the assumption will be correct.

When an abortion is performed by an experienced physician, with the observance of the utmost cleanliness (asepsis and antisepsis), then the abortion is accompanied with very little or no danger; but when performed carelessly, by incompetent, non-conscientious physicians and midwives, the operation is fraught with great danger to the patient's health or to her very life. And abortion is a great cause of premature death and chronic invalidism among women. And as long as the people will remain ignorant of the proper means of regulating their offspring, so long will abortion thrive.

While I recognize that there are cases in which the performance of an abortion is perfectly justifiable from a moral standpoint, for instance in cases of rape or where the mother is unmarried, nevertheless abortion must be recognized as an evil, a necessary evil now and then, but an evil, nevertheless. It is never to be undertaken lightly, or to be considered in a frivolous spirit; and it is the duty of all serious-minded and humanitarian men and women to do everything in their power to remove those conditions which make abortion necessary and unavoidable.

CHAPTER XVII

PRENATAL CARE

Meaning of the Term—Misleading Information by Quasi-Scientists—
Exaggerated Ideas Regarding Prenatal Care—Nervous Connection Between
Mother and Child—Cases Under Author's Observation—Effects on
Offspring—Advice to Pregnant Women—Germ-plasm of Chronic Alcoholic—
A Glass of Wine and the Spermatozoa—False Statements—Cases of Violence
and Accidents During Pregnancy.

By prenatal care we understand the care taken during pregnancy
before the child is born. Used in a wider sense the term includes the
care which both parents should take of themselves even before the
child is conceived.

Of course the father and the mother should be in the best possible
physical and mental condition during the time of conception and
even before conception, and the mother should take the very best
care of herself—she should be in good health and as calm a spirit as
possible during the entire period of gestation. For the general health
and condition of the mother does influence the child.

And still I feel impelled to say something which may meet with
violent opposition in some quarters. The trouble is, there are too
many half-baked scientists in our midst. They spread misleading
information and the public at large is too apt to take every statement
that has a quasi-scientific seal for something absolute, for something
positive, for something that admits of no exceptions.

I have seen so much misery caused by wrong prenatal care teaching
and by the foolish, exaggerated ideas on the subject, that I consider
it my duty to say something in order to counteract those erroneous
notions. I consider it my special mission to destroy error, mysticism
and superstition. And the prenatal care teaching as imparted by some
unfortunately partakes of all three of the above.

Of course, I repeat, the mother should try to be in the best possible condition while she is carrying the child. Nevertheless, it is foolish to imagine if the mother is not quite well, or is worried about something, or has a fit of anger, that it is invariably going to be reflected on the child. The child, as we know, has no nervous connection whatever with the mother, and it is only very violent or prolonged shocks that are apt to have an injurious influence.

I know of children that were carried by their mothers in anger and in anguish from the day of conception to the day of delivery. And still they were born perfectly normal. I know of a child whose mother was suffering the most hellish tortures of jealousy during the entire period of pregnancy, and still the child was born perfectly healthy, perfectly normal, and is now a splendid specimen of manhood. I know children whose mothers went through severe attacks of pneumonia, typhoid fever, etc., and still they were born perfectly healthy and perfectly normal. I know children whose mothers were using every means to abort them, took all kinds of internal medicines until they were deathly sick, and still they were born perfectly healthy and normal. I know children whose mothers tried to abort them by mechanical means, who went to abortionists who made one or more attempts to induce the abortion—I know even cases where the mothers bled as a result of such attempts—and nevertheless, the children were born perfectly healthy, developed normally physically and mentally.

Of course these are not things that I would advise women to do or to undergo. I would not advise pregnant women to worry, to be sick, to take poisonous medicines or to make attempts at abortion, but I merely bring up these points to emphasize to my readers not to take the necessity of prenatal care in too absolute a sense, and not to worry themselves unnecessarily if the conditions during their pregnancy are not all that could be desired. The child is not necessarily going to be affected. The condition of the germ-plasms, i.e., the condition of the ovum and the spermatozoa at the time of conception is more important than all subsequent care during gestation.

As there are foolish people who possess a peculiar knack of misinterpreting and misunderstanding everything, I wish to emphasize that hygiene during pregnancy should not be neglected. Everything possible should be done to put the mother in the best possible physical and mental condition. All I want to say is that it is bad to be insane on the subject, that it is bad to take things in an absolute sense, and that it is bad to exaggerate.

You will often hear it said that a child that was conceived when the father was in an exhilarated condition is apt to be epileptic, or nervous, or insane, and what not. This is also to be taken with a grain of salt. A chronic alcoholic has a defective germ-plasm, and his children are apt to be defective. But a glass of wine at a wedding banquet cannot affect the previously formed spermatozoa. And the statements about children being born defective or developing defectively because their fathers took an occasional glass of wine are unworthy of serious consideration; are unworthy of any consideration.

In connection with the above the reports of some cases of *violence* and *accidents* during pregnancy which, in spite of their severity, did not affect the children, will prove of interest.

A delicate little woman missed her periods. She was sure she couldn't be more than two weeks over-due. And this is what she did. For five nights in succession she took hot mustard baths and she took them so hot that each time she nearly fainted and came out from them like a broiled lobster. No effect. She then took a box of pills which cost her two dollars. No effect except causing diarrhea. She then took two boxes of capsules which upset her stomach and made her fearfully nauseous. No other effect. She then ate one-half a colocynth, which made her terribly sick, causing a bloody diarrhea. She had to stay in bed for three or four days. She then took burning vaginal injections with some ipecac in them. No effect except making her feel raw so that she needed large amounts of cold cream. She then took secale cornutum and radix gossypii. No effect except giving her a headache, making her sick to her stomach and completely destroying her appetite, so that within a very short time she lost nearly ten pounds. She was then told that long walks might be efficient. She took walks of six and seven miles at a time, coming home more dead than alive. No effect. She then heard that jumping off a table is a very efficient means. She did it a dozen times in succession so that she was completely fagged out and out of breath. Eight and a half months later she gave birth to a perfectly healthy, well-formed boy weighing eight pounds.

The following case was reported by Brillaud-Laujardiere. A farmer who was responsible for the condition of a servant of his household conceived the idea of riding horseback with her in order to bring about an abortion, and pushing her off when the horse was running at great speed. This he repeated several times. The woman gave birth to a perfectly normal infant at full term.

Hofmann reports that another farmer, under similar circumstances, brutally kicked the woman in the abdomen repeatedly until she lost consciousness. The pregnancy continued to full term notwithstanding. In another case of Hofmann's, a woman allowed a heavy door to fall upon her, but the pregnancy was not affected.

Dr. Guibout relates that a German woman, living with her husband in California, being pregnant, wished to return to Munich, her home-town, to be delivered. The train in which she travelled through Panama collided with another train. Threatened abortion required her to take a rest. She took a steamer and after a very rough passage reached Portsmouth. From there she went to Paris. Here she fell down a flight of stairs in the hotel where she was stopping. Again she was threatened with abortion, but after a rest was in good condition and continued her journey. She finally reached home, and was delivered at full term of a normal infant.

Vibert reports the case of a woman who was in a train accident which injured her severely, killed two of her children, but did not affect her pregnancy. She was delivered at the proper time of a normal baby.

CHAPTER XVIII

THE MENOPAUSE OR CHANGE OF LIFE

Time of Menopause—Cause of Suffering During Menopause—Reproductive Function and Sexual Function Not Synonymous—Increased Libido During Menopause—Change of Life in Men.

In the chapter on menstruation I referred briefly to the menopause. I will consider it here somewhat more in detail.

The menopause, also called the climacteric, and in common language "change of life," is the period at which woman ceases to menstruate. The average age at which this occurs is about forty-eight. But while some women continue to menstruate up to the age of fifty, fifty-two, and even fifty-five, others cease to menstruate at the age of forty-five or even forty-two. Between forty-four and fifty-two are the normal limits. Anything before or beyond that is exceptional.

Just as the beginning of menstruation may set in without any trouble of any kind, and just as some women have not the slightest unpleasant symptoms during the entire period of their menstrual life, so the menopause occurs in some women without any trouble, physical or psychic. The periods between the menses become perhaps a little longer, or a little irregular, the menstrual flow becomes more and more scanty, then one or several periods may be skipped altogether, and the menopause is permanently established. Many women, however, the majority probably, suffer considerably during the transitional year or years of the menopause. Symptoms are both of a physical and of a psychic character, but the psychic symptoms predominate. There may be headache, capricious appetite, or complete loss of appetite, considerable loss of flesh, or on the contrary very sudden and rapid putting on of fat, great irritability, insomnia, profuse perspiration; hot flashes throughout the body, and particularly in the face, which make the face "blushing" and congested, are particularly frequent. Then the woman's character may be completely changed. From gentle and submissive she may become pugnacious and quarrelsome. Jealousy without any grounds for it may be one of the disagreeable symptoms, making both the wife and the husband very unhappy. In some exceptional cases a genuine neurosis or psychosis may develop.

Cause of Suffering During Menopause. It is my conviction, and I have had this conviction for many years, that many, if not most, of the distressing symptoms of the menopause are due, not to the menopause itself, but to the wrong ideas about this period that have prevailed for so many centuries. We know the influence of the mind over the body, and the pernicious effect which wrong ideas may exercise over our feelings. The generally prevalent opinion among women, and men for that matter, and not only of the laity but unfortunately of the medical profession as well, is that the menopause is the end of woman's sexual life. Every woman is laboring under the erroneous impression that with the establishment of the menopause, with the cessation of the menses, she ceases to be a woman, and as she does not become a man, she becomes something of a neuter being, neither woman nor man. And she has the idea that after the menopause she can have no further attraction for her husband or for other men. Naturally such an idea has a very depressing effect on any human being. Any human being fights to the last to retain all its human functions, especially the function which is considered as important as is the sexual function.

Reproductive Function and Sexual Function Not Synonymous. Of course with the permanent cessation of the menses the woman's *reproductive* function is at an end. But the reproductive function is *not* synonymous with the sexual function, I must insist again and again, and naturally until this erroneous idea is dispelled much unnecessary misery will be the lot of our women. If women in general will learn that with the establishment of the menopause they do *not* cease to be women, if they will learn that the sexual desire in women lasts long beyond the cessation of the menopause, many women being as passionate at sixty as at thirty, if they will learn that their attractiveness or non-attractiveness to the male sex does not depend upon the menopause, but upon their general condition, if they will learn that many women at fifty and sixty are much more attractive than some women at half that age, they will not take the onset of the menopause so tragically and they will thereby avoid the greater part of their mental and emotional suffering.

The actual atrophy of the ovaries, uterus, external genitals and the breasts can, of course, not be prevented, but that atrophy is a slow and gradual process, and is not in itself the cause of the various distressing symptoms that we have enumerated.

The treatment of the menopause, if the symptoms are at all disagreeable, or distressing, should be in the hands of a competent physician. A little wholesome advice may be more efficient than gallons of medicine and bushels of pills. In general the woman should try to lead as calm and peaceful a life as possible. Warm baths daily are beneficial, constipation should be guarded against, hot vaginal douches are often efficient against the disagreeable flushes, and last, but not least, the husband should during this critical period be doubly kind and doubly considerate of his wife. It is during the years between forty-five and fifty-five that the wife is most in need of her husband's sympathy and support.

Increased Libido During Menopause. There is one rather delicate symptom which I must not pass unmentioned. Some women during the years while the menopause is being established, and for some years after the menopause, experience a greatly heightened sexual desire. In some cases this increased libido is normal, that is, no other pathologic symptoms or local conditions can be discovered. In some cases the increased libido is distinctly due to local congestion, congestion of the ovaries, the uterus, etc. In some cases, I can distinctly testify, it is psychic or autosuggestive. Because the woman thinks, and believes that other people think, that she is soon going to lose all her sexuality, she unconsciously works herself up into a sexual passion which sometimes may be of long duration and may even lead to disastrous results.

What to do in such cases? Where the woman's libido is normal or near normal, then naturally it should be normally gratified. But if the libido seems to be abnormally strong and the demands for sexual gratification are too frequent, then the woman should be treated and sexual gratification should not be indulged in, because in such cases, as a rule, sexual gratification only adds fuel to the fire, and the woman's demands may become more and more frequent, more and more insistent. In exceptional cases it may even reach the intensity of nymphomania. In such cases the aid of a tactful physician is indispensable.

CHANGE OF LIFE IN MEN

To people not familiar with the subject it sounds rather strange to speak of "change of life" in men.

Man, possessing no menstrual function, cannot have any menopause, but still sexologists and psychologists who have studied the subject carefully are convinced that between the ages of forty-five and fifty-five men also undergo a certain change which may be spoken of as the change of life or the male climacteric.

They become irritable, capricious, very susceptible to feminine charms, are apt to fall in love, and in many the sexual instinct is greatly increased. As in women, this increase of the sexual desire is sometimes due to pathologic causes, such as an inflamed prostate gland—in other cases it is of psychic origin.

Just as a man should be particularly kind and considerate to his wife during her menopause, so the wife, understanding that her husband is going through a critical period, will also increase her tact, patience and consideration.

CHAPTER XIX

THE HABIT OF MASTURBATION

Definition of Masturbation—Its Injurious Effects in Girls as Compared with Boys—Married Life of the Girl Masturbator—Necessity for Change in Injurious Attitude of Parents who Discover the Habit—Common-sense Treatment of the Habit—How to Prevent Formation of Habit—Parents' Advice to Children—Hot Baths as Factor in Masturbation—Other Physical Factors— Mental Masturbation and Its Effects.

Masturbation or self-abuse is a term applied to a bad habit which consists in handling and rubbing the genitals. It is a bad habit because it is apt to injure the health and future development of the girl. The more frequently it is practiced, the more injurious it is. It is more injurious than when practiced by boys, because the effects are usually more permanent. Girls who indulge in the habit of masturbation to excess not only weaken themselves, become anemic and get a dingy, pimply complexion, but they lose their desire for normal sexual relations when they grow up, and are unable to derive any pleasure from the sexual act when they get married. In fact, many girls who masturbated excessively get a strong aversion to the normal sexual act, and their married life is an unhappy one. Their husbands often have to ask for a divorce. Fortunately, the habit is much less widespread among girls than it is among boys. While about ninety per cent. of all boys—nine out of every ten— masturbate more or less, only about ten or at most twenty per cent. of girls are addicted to this habit. But whatever the percentage may be, the habit is an injurious one, and if you value your health, your beauty and proper growth and mental development, you should not indulge in it. If you are already indulging, if you are used to handling your genitals, if a bad companion has initiated you into the habit, you should give it up. And mothers should watch their children, guard them against developing the habit, and do everything possible to cure them of it, if prevention comes too late.

But while as you see I do not deny the evil effects of masturbation, it is necessary to state that a great change has taken place in our opinions on the subject, and it is but right that parents should know of this change of opinion among the medical profession, particularly among those who specialize in sexology.

Wrong Behavior of Parents. When parents make the "awful" discovery that their child is fondling its genitals or is indulging in masturbation, they feel as if a great calamity had befallen them. They could not feel worse if they learned that the child was a thief or a pyromaniac. Imbued with the medieval idea of the "sinfulness" of the habit, as well as its injuriousness, they begin to scold the child, to frighten it, to make it believe that it is doing something terrible, that it has disgraced them and itself; and they try to persuade it that, unless it stops immediately, the most direful consequences are awaiting it. The results of this mode of procedure are disastrous— much more so than is the masturbation itself.

Often the scolding and the exposure of the child are done in the presence of others. This implants in the poor girl a sullen resentment that only makes it more difficult for it to break the habit. When the child is brought to the physician, you can see by its behavior, by its downcast looks, by its sulkiness, by its attempt to refrain from tears, and other signs, that it regards the physician in exactly the same light as a youthful criminal regards the judge before whom he has been brought for trial.

It is time, high time, that this silly and injurious attitude toward a practice, which is very common, be radically changed. It is time that parents and physicians learn that the injuriousness of the habit has been greatly, grossly exaggerated. It is time that they know that the vast majority of boys and girls get over the habit without being much, or any, the worse for it. The knowledge of this fact will not only save them and the children much needless anguish and suffering, but will make it much easier to deal with the latter, make it much easier to get them divorced from the habit.

If we look at the matter in a sensible, common-sense way, and do not tell the child caught in the practice that it has done something disgracefully vicious and criminal, but speak to it kindly and tell it that it is doing something that may injure it greatly, that may interfere with its future mental and physical health and development, then we shall have far greater success in our endeavors to break the boy or the girl of the habit of masturbation. As I have said in another place:

"In my opinion, stigmatizing even the most moderate indulgence in masturbation as a vice has a deleterious effect upon the people who so indulge and makes it harder for them to break off the habit. Every thinking physician and sexologist can tell you that picturing the masturbatory habit in too lurid colors and stigmatizing it with too strong epithets has, as a rule, the contrary effect to the one expected. The victims of the habit consider themselves degraded, irretrievably lost. They lose their self-respect, and it is, on account of that, harder for them to break themselves of the habit."

We shall accomplish a good deal more with our youthful and older patients if we leave alone, altogether, the moral side of the question—if there be any moral side to it—and emphasize the physical injuriousness of the habit. We do not want to diminish the self-respect of our boys and girls, we want to increase it; and we can not do this if we make them believe that a masturbator is a vicious criminal. Inspire your patients with confidence, tell them that indulgence in the habit jeopardizes their future growth, both physical and mental, their health and happiness, and you will find them easier to control.

I am not trying to minimize the danger of masturbation, for, if indulged in from an early age and to great excess, the results *may* be disastrous. But, even if I were to minimize the evil consequences, that would be less of a sin than to exaggerate them the way it has been done for so many years, by so many people in the profession and out of it. The evil results of exaggerating the influence of masturbation have been so great in the past that, if now the pendulum were to swing to the other extreme, I am sure it would not be a bad thing at all.

To deal with the subject of the *treatment* of masturbation belongs to a medical treatise. But, a few remarks on how to prevent children from acquiring the habit of masturbation will not be out of place.

Prevention of the Habit of Masturbation. The keynote of preventing the habit is, carefully to watch the child from its earliest infancy. We know that not infrequently stupid or vicious nursemaids, wet-nurses, and even governesses ignorantly or deliberately induce the habit in children under their charge. This, of course, must be prevented. Even children of the age of nine, ten, eleven years should not be left alone, but always be under supervision. Too close friendship between boys or girls, particularly of different ages, should be looked upon with suspicion.

A number of girls never should sleep in the same room without supervision by an older person.

The sleeping together of two in the same bed, whether it be two children or a grown person and a child, should not be permitted under any circumstances. I admit of no exceptions to this demand. It makes no difference whether the other person is a mother, a father, a brother or a sister. Leaving out of the question any *deliberate* element, the thing is dangerous; for, very often, unintentionally, unwittingly, masturbation is initiated by this intimate contact.

The child—boy or girl—should sleep alone, on a rather hard mattress. The covering should be light. A coverlet may be put over the feet. The child always should sleep with the arms out upon the cover or blanket, never *under* the same. If this is done from childhood on, it is very easy to get used to this way of sleeping, and many a case of masturbation will thus be obviated. The child should not be permitted to loll in bed: it must be taught to get up as soon as it awakes in the morning. The general bringing-up must be of a strengthening, hardening character; and this applies both to the body and the will. When the children reach the age of nine, ten, eleven, twelve or thirteen years (we must use discrimination and judgment, for, some children of nine are as developed as are others of thirteen), we must tell them that it is bad and injurious to handle one's genitals, and we must warn them to shun any companions who wish to initiate them into any manipulations of these parts or who show an inclination to talk about the sexual organs and sex matters.

Hot baths are very injurious for young children in their influence in this direction. There is no question that a hot bath has a very decided stimulating effect upon the sexual desire of adults as well as of children, both male and female; in fact, I have had several patients of either sex tell me that their first masturbatory act was committed while they were in a hot bath. Of course, the sensation having been pleasurable, they kept on repeating the experience.

Every factor liable to give rise to the habit should be removed. Thus, for instance, eczema about the genitals, strongly acid urine, seatworms, and the like, should be treated until cured. That anything having a tendency prematurely to awaken the sexual instinct should be rigorously avoided, goes without saying.

Mental or Psychic Masturbation. Some girls and women will abstain from handling themselves with their hands (manual masturbation), but will practice what we call mental masturbation. That is, they will concentrate their minds on the opposite sex, will picture to themselves various lascivious scenes, until they feel "satisfied." This method is extremely injurious and exhausting and is very likely to lead to neurasthenia and a nervous breakdown. You should break yourself of it, by all means, if you can. For it is even more injurious than the regular habit.

CHAPTER XX

LEUCORRHEA—THE WHITES

Misconception Regarding the Meaning of the Term "Leucorrhea"—A Common Complaint—Severe Cases—Reasons for Resistance to Treatment—Proper Local Treatment of the Disorder—Sterility Due to Leucorrhea—Causes of Leucorrhea—Tonic Medicines—Local Treatment—Formulæ for Douching.

Leucorrhea means literally a "white running," and is applied by the laity to any whitish discharge coming from the vagina. This is wrong, because some white discharges may be of little importance; others may be of a serious character, and not be leucorrhea at all.

Leucorrhea is one of the banes of the modern girl and woman. It is very frequent. Probably at least twenty-five per cent, (some say fifty or seventy-five per cent.) of all women suffer with it in a greater or lesser degree. In some cases it is only an annoyance, necessitating the frequent changing of napkins, but in others it causes a great deal of weakness, backache, erosions, itching and burning. It is very resistant to treatment, particularly in girls. The reason it is so resistant to treatment is because the discharge, while coming from the vagina, *does not usually originate* in the vagina; it originates in the neck of the womb, and the hundreds and hundreds of injections that women take for their leucorrhea only reach the vagina; they cannot penetrate into the womb. And it is only by treating the cavity of the cervix, which can only be done by a physician, through a speculum, that the root of the trouble can be reached. And, if any erosion or ulcer is noticed, it can be directly touched up with the necessary application. And it is for this reason that in girls leucorrhea is so much more difficult to treat. For fear of having the hymen ruptured the girl objects to a thorough examination and to local treatment, and the leucorrhea is permitted to proceed until perhaps a chronic inflammation of the womb and the Fallopian tubes is established. There is no doubt that many cases of sterility or childlessness in women are due to long-neglected leucorrhea in girlhood.

What Is the Cause of Leucorrhea? We can answer simply: the cause of leucorrhea is catarrh in any part of the female genital tract. But this is no real answer. What are the causes of the catarrh? The causes of catarrh are many: the most common cause is a cold. Wetting the feet and getting chilled, particularly during the menses, may set up a catarrh in the cervix. Long standing on one's feet, lifting and carrying heavy bundles, dancing in overheated rooms and then going out scantily clad in the chill night air, prolonged ungratified sexual excitement, lack of cleanliness in the external genitals—all these are factors in setting up a catarrh of the cervix with a resultant leucorrhea. A general rundown condition, worry, overwork, too hard study, lack of fresh air, and a general scrofulous condition also favor the development of catarrh of the womb and leucorrhea. It will therefore be seen that the treatment of leucorrhea to be successful must be general and local.

General Treatment. The general treatment consists in general hygienic measures and in common sense. The patient should not be on her feet more than she can help, and she should not walk until exhausted or fatigued. It is better to take several short walks than one long one. The corset she wears, if she wears any at all, should be of the modern kind: not one that presses the womb and the other abdominal organs down, but one that supports the abdominal walls, and rather raises the abdominal organs up. The lacing or buttoning must be from below up, and not from above down. That it should not in any way interfere with the freedom of respiration goes without saying. Constipation if any, to be treated, must be treated intelligently, by mild measures (see **Constipation**, in the chapter on pregnancy), and care must be taken that the bowels move at regular hours. Where the leucorrhea is due to or is aggravated by anemia and general weakness, a good iron preparation, such as one Blaud's five-grain pill three times a day, or a tonic of iron, quinine and strychnine, will do good. A daily cold bath or cold sponge, followed by a brisk dry rubbing with a rough towel, is also useful.

Local Treatment. Local measures consist of painting or swabbing the vagina and cervix with various solutions, of tampons, suppositories and douches. Local application to the vagina and uterus can be done satisfactorily by the physician or nurse only. The insertion of a suppository or douching can be easily done by the patient herself.

While it is always best and safest to consult a physician, and, while self-medication is generally inadvisable, there are occasions when a physician is not available; in some small places a woman may, *for various reasons*, have a strong objection to gynecological examination and treatment; and some women may be too poor to pay the doctor. In such circumstances self-treatment is justified and there can be no objection to it if the remedies are harmless and are sure to do some good; that is, to improve the condition where they do not effect a complete cure.

One of the simplest things is an alum tampon. You take a piece of absorbent cotton, about the size of a fist, spread it out, put about a tablespoonful of powdered alum on it, fold it up, tie a string around the center, insert it in the vagina as far as it will go, and leave it in for twenty-four hours. Then pull it gently by the string and syringe yourself with a quart or two quarts of warm water. Such a tampon may be inserted every other day or every third day, and I have known many cases where this simple treatment alone produced a cure. In some cases, however, douches work better and the two best things for douching are: tincture of iodine and lactic acid. Buy, say, four ounces of tincture of iodine, and use two teaspoonfuls in two quarts of hot water in a douche bag. This injection should be used twice a day, morning and night. Of the lactic acid you buy, say, a pint, and use two tablespoonfuls to two quarts of water. The lactic acid has the advantage over the tincture of iodine that it is colorless, while the iodine is dark and stains whatever it comes in contact with. Sometimes I order the use of the tincture of iodine and the lactic acid alternately: for one douche the tincture of iodine, for the next the lactic acid, and so on. When the condition improves, it is sufficient to use one teaspoonful of the tincture of iodine and one tablespoonful of the lactic acid to two quarts of water. These injections are quite efficient and have the advantage of being perfectly harmless. One point about the injections: they should be taken not in the standing or squatting position (in which position the fluid comes right out), but while lying down, over a douche pan. The douche bag should be only about a foot above the bed, so that the irrigating fluid may come out slowly; the patient, after each injection taken in the daytime, should remain at least half an hour in bed (in the night time she stays all night in bed). This gives the injection a better chance to come in contact with all the parts of the vagina, and a portion of it comes in contact with the cervix, where it exerts a healing effect. Avoid the use of patent medicines.

CHAPTER XXI

THE VENEREAL DISEASES

Derivation of Word "Venereal"—Three Venereal Diseases—Innocent Contraction of Syphilis Through Various Objects—The Hygienic Elimination of Common Sources of Venereal Infection—Measures for Prevention After Sexual Relations.

The word "venereal" means pertaining to sexual intercourse: venereal excess—excess in sexual intercourse; venereal disease—a disease acquired from sexual intercourse with an infected person. The word is derived from Venus (genitive—veneris), the Roman goddess of spring, flowers and Love.

There are three venereal diseases: gonorrhea, syphilis and chancroid. Of these, gonorrhea is the most widespread, syphilis the most serious. Chancroid is of comparatively little importance.

While by far the greatest amount of venereal diseases—probably ninety per cent, of the total—is contracted from illicit intercourse,[7] it is well to bear in mind that some of it is contracted innocently, either from a kiss, or from using a sponge or a towel which has been used by an infected person, etc. While the gonorrheal germ is generally transmitted directly, the syphilitic poison may be transmitted through various objects. Syphilis contracted not during intercourse, but in an innocent manner, from a kiss, a towel, a toothbrush, a razor, etc., is called syphilis of the innocent, or syphilis insontium. In former years doctors would not very rarely contract syphilis from examining syphilitic women with their bare fingers. Now since gloves have come into use for examining purposes, the number of infections has considerably diminished. And no doubt that as the people become more familiar with the danger of venereal infection from non-venereal sources, the number of innocent infections will greatly diminish. The dangerous roller towel and the

---

[7] Illicit—illegal, non-permissible, outside of marriage.

no less dangerous common drinking cup are being gradually eliminated as factors of *non-venereal* infection; and we may confidently expect that in a decade or two the amount of venereal disease from *venereal* infection will be greatly lessened in all civilized countries. The general increase in cleanliness in all strata of society and the universal use of antiseptics after suspicious sexual relations will constitute the chief factors in this diminution of venereal disease.

CHAPTER XXII

THE EXTENT OF VENEREAL DISEASE

Former Ban on Discussion of Venereal Disease and Its Evil Results—Present Reprehensible Exaggerations of Extent of Venereal Disease—Erroneous and Ridiculous Statements of "Reformers"—Senseless Fear of Marriage in Girls Due to Lurid Exaggerations—Study by Woman Psychologist Reveals Harmful Results of Exaggerated Statements—Truth in Regard to Percentage of Men Afflicted with Venereal Disease.

Former Silence. Only a very few years ago respectable women, by which I mean all women outside of the women called "fallen," did not know of the existence of venereal disease. It was considered a prohibited, disgraceful subject, not to be mentioned or even hinted at in conversation, in books or magazines, in lectures, or on the stage. When I say that they did not know of the *existence* of such a thing as venereal disease, that the very words gonorrhea and syphilis were unknown to them, I use these expressions not as figures of speech, but in their literal meaning. All avenues of acquiring such knowledge being closed to them—lay people don't usually now and they surely didn't then purchase and read strictly medical works—where could they obtain the information? The result was that when a woman was so unfortunate as to contract a venereal disease from her husband, she did not understand its character and did not suspect its source. Which was a rather good thing—for the husband. Family peace was more secure.

Present Exaggerations. Now a change has taken place in this respect, and, as is often the case with recent changes, the pendulum has swung to the other extreme. The silence of former days has given place to shouting from the housetops. The last phrase is also used almost in its literal sense. Many men and women, deeply stirred by the venereal peril, and sincerely anxious to guard boys and girls from venereal infection, have been indulging in very reprehensible exaggerations. Particularly lurid have been the exaggerations as to the prevalence of the disease in the male sex, with its consequent disastrous effects on married women. A statement made by a Dr.

Noeggerath (a German physician who practiced at the time in New York), nearly half a century ago, to the effect that 80 per cent, of all men have gonorrhea and that 90 per cent. of these remain uncured and infect or are apt to infect their wives, has been shown to be a ridiculously absurd exaggeration. If it had been true, the race would now be at the point of dying out. Nevertheless, this statement is copied from book to book, as if it were gospel truth, as if it were a scientifically and statistically established fact instead of a wild, sensational guess. An esteemed New York physician, Dr. Prince A. Morrow, did excellent pioneer work in calling attention to the dangers of venereal disease. But, as is the case with so many "reformers," he permitted his zeal to run away with him occasionally, and he made statements which caused and are still causing the judicious to grieve. The statement, for instance, that there is more venereal disease among innocent, virtuous wives than among prostitutes is one to cause the real honest investigator to weep (over the human tendency to exaggeration), or to burst out in uproarious laughter. The ridiculousness of this statement becomes especially evident when we recollect that the same gentleman made the statement that every prostitute, without exception, was diseased at one time or another. If venereal disease exists among prostitutes to the extent of 100 per cent., then how can it exist to a greater extent among innocent, virtuous wives? And to still further emphasize the absurdity of the above statement, I will tell you that the extent of venereal disease among married women is believed by careful non-sensational venereologists not to exceed five per cent.!

Yes, the silence of former years has given place to the lurid exaggeration of the present day. While on the whole the former was worse than the latter, the latter is bad enough, because it makes many girls unhappy, sowing in them the seeds of suspicion and cynicism, tends to make them antagonistic to the entire male sex, and inoculates them with a senseless fear of marriage. A study made by Miriam C. Gould, of the department of psychology and philosophy in the University of Pittsburg (*Social Hygiene*, April, 1916), corroborates our remarks in a striking manner.

She has had confidential chats with 50 young girls, with whom she has had some acquaintance; of these 50, 25 were college students and 25 were not. She asked them a number of questions, the purpose of which was to find out what psychologic effect, if any, their knowledge of prostitution and of venereal disease has had on them. She states in her conclusions that "the histories reveal a large percentage of harmful results, such as conditions bordering upon neurasthenia, melancholia, pessimism and *sex antagonism* (italics mine), directly traceable to this knowledge. Eleven of the girls interviewed developed a pronounced repulsion for men, although prior to their 'knowledge' they had enjoyed men's company. They now avoid association with them, and six have declared that they have totally lost faith in the moral cleanness of men. Eight have already refused to marry, or intend to do so, because of their belief that the risk of infection was too great. If it were not for the existence of these diseases, they say they would be glad to marry. All of these say their decision has rendered them more or less unhappy."

In the laudable desire to keep our young women pure and to protect them from infection, in the endeavor to make them demand one moral standard for both sexes, our exaggerating reformers are condemning them to lifelong celibacy, which in the case of women often means lifelong neurasthenia and hypochondria.

The Truth of the Matter. Here is the Truth about venereal disease—the truth as I know it, without concealment on the one hand and without exaggeration on the other. Exact figures are, of course, unobtainable anywhere; but results obtained from unbiased investigations of *different* classes of society, from hospital reports, from questionnaires among students, etc., tell us that probably about twenty per cent. of the adult male population are the victims of gonorrhea at one time or another; that probably eight or ten per cent. are not entirely cured when they enter matrimony; and four or five per cent. (some would say two per cent.) of wives become infected with gonorrhea. This, I say, is terrible enough, and makes the greatest care and caution imperative; for, if you should be one of the victims of the two or five per cent., it would be little consolation to you that the other ninety-eight or ninety-five per cent. of wives have escaped.

Of course the percentage of venereal disease among young men, and afterwards among their wives, will vary greatly with the stratum of society. Among the "lower" strata you may find fifty per cent. of infection, with a very large percentage of those uncured. Not because they are of a lower morality than the higher classes, but because the cheap class of prostitutes that they are obliged to patronize are frequently diseased and because they cannot afford expert treatment, or any treatment at all. Among these classes you will naturally find a much larger percentage of diseased wives. But then to counteract this we must bear in mind that there are large classes of men in whom gonorrhea exists only to the extent of five or ten per cent., and we have large classes of wives among whom the victims of gonorrhea will come up only to a fraction of one per cent.

The above figures, you see, differ materially from the statements found in so many sex books that "80 per cent. of all married men in New York have gonorrhea," and that "at least three out of every five per cent.! married women in New York have gonorrhea." Whenever you read or hear such a statement treat it with a smile—or with contempt, as all false statements should be treated.

As to syphilis, the extent of the prevalence may be given as between two and five per cent. Which percentage differs considerable from the 75, 50 or 25 per cent. given us by some sex lecturers, but which is terrible enough as it is, without any exaggerations.

CHAPTER XXIII

GONORRHEA

Source of Gonorrhea—Mucous Membrane of Genital Organs and of Eye Principal Seats of Disease—Symptoms in Men and in Women—Vagina Seldom Attacked in Adults—Nobody Inherits Gonorrhea—Ophthalmia Neonatorum—Differences of Course of Disease in Men and Women—Gonorrhea Less Painful in Women—Symptoms not Suspected by Woman—Necessity for the Woman Consulting a Physician—Self-treatment When Woman Cannot Consult Physician—Formulæ for Injections.

The subject of gonorrhea and syphilis is treated pretty fully, from a layman's point of view, in the author's *Sex Knowledge for Men*. I do not intend to devote much space to a discussion of the details of these two diseases here, because the subject is not of such direct interest to women. Respectable girls and women do not indulge in illicit relations the same as respectable men and boys do, and their danger of contracting a venereal disease is insignificant as compared with men's liability. I will, therefore, touch upon only a few points, particularly insofar as the diseases differ in their course from the

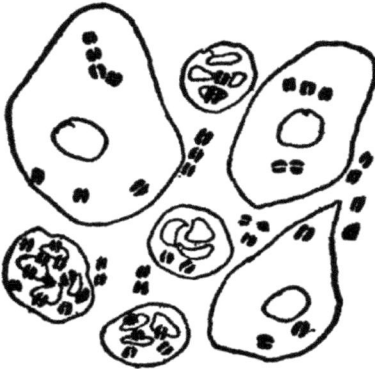

course pursued in men. Those, however, who are interested may read the chapters on the subject in the author's *Sex Knowledge for Men*, and if they want still fuller details, they may study the author's *Treatment of Gonorrhea and Its Complications in Men and Women*.

Gonorrheal Germs.

Gonorrhea is an inflammation caused by a germ called the gonococcus, discovered by Dr. A. Neisser, of Breslau, Germany, in 1879. Any mucous membrane may be the seat of gonorrhea, but it attacks by preference the mucous membrane of the genital organs, and of one other organ—the eye. Its principal symptoms are: inflammation, pain, burning and discharge. In men, it attacks the urethra; in women it attacks the cervix—the neck of the womb—the urethra, and the vulva. The vagina is seldom attacked in adult women, because the mucous membrane of the adult vagina is rather tough and does not offer a good soil for the development of the gonococcus germ. The discharge that a woman has when she has gonorrhea comes principally or exclusively from the neck of the womb. In little girls, however, in whom the lining of the vagina is tender, gonorrhea of the vagina and the vulva is common. (See chapter **Vulvovaginitis in Little Girls.**) Gonorrhea is a local disease. While in some cases, after the disease has lasted for some time, a certain poison is generated by the germs which circulates in the blood, and while the germs may occasionally wander into distant organs, still in 98 per cent. of all cases gonorrhea is a local disease, and if taken in time is cured without leaving any traces on the general organism.

Gonorrhea Not Hereditary. Then, gonorrhea is not a hereditary disease. Nobody ever *inherits* gonorrhea. A child may be born with a gonorrheal inflammation of the eyes (ophthalmia neonatorum), but this inflammation is not inherited; it can only be acquired if the mother is suffering with gonorrhea while the child is being born: some of the pus in the mother's birth canal gets into the child's eyes while it passes through the uterus and vagina. This is not heredity; this is simple infection, and can be avoided by keeping the mother's birth canal clean by antiseptic douches before childbirth. In short, I repeat gonorrhea is essentially a local and not a constitutional disease, and is not hereditary. In which two respects it differs from syphilis, which is the most constitutional and most hereditary of all diseases.

Course of Gonorrhea in Men and Women. Gonorrhea runs an entirely different course in women than it does in men. When a man has gonorrhea he knows it immediately; first, because the discharge tells him that there is something the matter with him, for a man is not used to having any discharge from the urethra unless there is something the matter with him. Second, the urine becomes at once burning and painful. In women the urethra is a separate canal from the vagina, and the urethra is very frequently not affected in gonorrhea. The infection generally starts in the cervix, and the disease may last for considerable time before the woman becomes aware of it. In general, gonorrhea is a less painful disease in woman, and this is a bad thing, because she thus neglects treatment and loses valuable time, permitting the disease to develop. Even when the urethra is affected in women, it does not give as severe symptoms as inflammation of the urethra in men. If the woman does have pains she often pays no attention to them, because woman is used to pains; as we have seen before, fifty per cent. of all women suffer more or less with dysmenorrhea. Many of them have a leucorrheal discharge of greater or lesser degree, and therefore if there is an increase in the pains, or an increase in the discharge, little attention is paid to the matter. In fact, a woman may have a chronic gonorrhea for months or years without being aware that there is anything the matter with her. It is important to teach women to seek medical aid as soon as they notice any increase in the amount of the discharge, or change in color, particularly if it becomes greenish, or if the odor becomes offensive, or if there is chafing, burning, or irritation around the genitals, and particularly if there is an increase in the frequency or urgency of urination, or if there is a burning, scalding, or cutting sensation during the act of urination. Also whenever the sexual act becomes painful. If women consulted a physician as soon as they noticed any of the symptoms referred to above, they would save months and years of suffering and expense, because the disease would often be taken in hand while still limited to the cervix, and not, as is now often the case, after the inflammation has extended into the uterus and Fallopian tubes.

Self-treatment. I do not believe in self-treatment because it is generally unsatisfactory and may often even become dangerous, and I decidedly advise every woman who suspects that she has contracted gonorrhea to apply at once to a competent physician. But it happens not infrequently that a woman is so situated that she cannot consult a physician. And in the meantime there is danger of the gonorrhea spreading further and further. In such cases it is advisable for the woman to use an injection until such time when she can consult a physician. The injection I am going to advise may in itself produce a cure; and, if it does not produce a complete cure, it at any rate improves the condition, prevents the extension of the disease, makes subsequent treatment easier, and besides is perfectly harmless. The best injection for self use in gonorrhea is tincture of iodine; the proportion is two teaspoonfuls to a quart or two quarts of water. If the case is very bad, such an injection may be taken twice a day. If the case is not very bad, once a day is sufficient. After using the tincture of iodine for five days to a week, it is good to change off to lactic acid. Buy a pint or so of lactic acid in a drug store, and use one tablespoonful to a quart of water. It is preferable to have the water hot, about 100 deg., but where this is inconvenient it may be used lukewarm. The lactic acid injection is used for three days, then the iodine injection is resumed, then again the lactic acid, and so on. I know of many cases that were cured by this treatment alone. And I might mention that these injections are generally also very efficient in leucorrhea, as stated in the chapter on Leucorrhea.

CHAPTER XXIV

VULVOVAGINITIS IN LITTLE GIRLS

Former Causes of Vulvovaginitis in Little Girls—Discharge Chief Symptom—
Evil Results of Vulvovaginitis—Psychic Results of Treatment—Effects in
Hastening Sexual Maturity—Vulvovaginitis a Cause of Permanent Sterility—
Measures to Prevent the Disease—Toilet Seats and Vulvovaginitis.

The mucous membrane, or the lining of the vulva and vagina, in little girls is very tender, and therefore very readily subject to infection. An infection of the vulva and vagina due to the gonococcus or to some other germ is very common in little girls. At least it used to be, particularly among children of the poor, in institutions and hospitals. The very dangerous infective character of vulvovaginitis was not known, and the infection was therefore easily transferred by towels, linen, toilet seats, bedpans, syringe nozzles, thermometers, the nurses' hands, and in various other ways. Now great care is being taken and in most hospitals no children are admitted in the general wards unless it is determined that they are free from vulvovaginitis.

Generally speaking, vulvovaginitis in children is a mild infection. A child may have it for several weeks or months without being aware of it, without saying anything about it, the diagnosis often being made by the mother, who begins to notice the creamy discharge on the girl's linen or underwear. And this is the principal symptom in little girls thus afflicted—the discharge. This discharge may be very profuse, covering the vulva, vagina, and cervix.

In severe cases, there is also an infection of the urethra, and the child may complain of burning at urination, itching and pain around the vulva and anus, and slight pain in the abdomen. There may be a moderate rise in temperature, up to 101 deg. F., and in some instances the attack is sufficiently acute to give rise to a chill and fever. A mild inflammation of the joints may set in within the first weeks of the infection, although as a usual thing it comes later on.

Evil Sequelæ of Vulvovaginitis. While, as stated, vulvovaginitis is a comparatively mild infection as far as its symptoms are concerned, it nevertheless has a very bad effect on the child who is unfortunate enough to become a victim of the disease. First of all, it is an extremely long drawn, persistent disease. It usually takes months, and these months may run into years, before a complete cure, is effected. Second, relapses are quite common. Third, the treatment is a disagreeable one for the child, and is occasionally painful. Fourth, it has a disastrous effect on the child's *morale*; most parents, though they may love the child most affectionately, look somewhat askance at it; and continuous vaginal treatment somehow or other has a humiliating effect on the child, which begins to consider itself as an outcast, as something apart from other children. Fifth, the child's education is very frequently seriously and permanently interfered with, because it must often be taken out of school, whether public or private, and private tutoring is of course feasible only for the few. Sixth, and this is a point not sufficiently appreciated by the profession and the laity, but it is an important point, nevertheless: vulvovaginitis in children has unfortunately a disastrous effect in *hastening the sexual maturity of the child*. Whether this is due to the congestion of the organs produced by the inflammation, or to the speculum examinations, paintings, douches, applications, tampons, suppositories, etc., the fact remains that girls who suffer from vulvovaginitis in childhood become sexually mature considerably earlier than normal girls of the same class, stratum and climate, and their demand for sexual satisfaction is much more insistent. Seventh, a mild vulvovaginitis may be the cause of permanent *sterility*.

It will therefore be seen that vulvovaginitis is a calamity, and everything possible should be done to guard female children from contracting it. *All* children should *always* sleep alone. Under no circumstances should a child sleep with anybody else, be it a sister, a mother, a friend, a governess, or a servant girl. People should be very careful in sending their children to spend a night or two with some friends. The friends may be all right, but still a friend of the friends or a relative of the friends may not be. I have known several cases where the origin of the vulvovaginitis could be traced to little girls spending a week at the house of some friends where a boarder or relative was infected with gonorrhea. That children should be kept away from associating or playing with adults or other children who are known to have gonorrheal infection goes without saying.

The child's genitals should be frequently inspected by the mother, and scrupulous cleanliness by frequent bathing, sponging with warm solutions and powdering, should be maintained. The toilet seats in school should receive special attention. The wooden seat is a menace because it often harbors gonorrheal pus from either the female or male genitals, while the only proper seat is one of the so-called U-shaped style, that is, one in which the front is entirely open, like the letter U.

CHAPTER XXV

SYPHILIS

Syphilis Due to Germ—Syphilis a Constitutional Disease—Primary Lesion—Incubation Period—Roseola—Primary Stage—Secondary Stage—Mucous Patches—Tertiary Stage—Gumma—Hereditary Nature of Syphilis—Milder Course in Women Than in Men—Obscure Symptoms in Syphilis—Necessity for Examination by Physician—Locomotor Ataxia—Softening of the Brain—Chancroids.

Syphilis is a disease caused by a germ called spirocheta; the full name is spirocheta pallida—a pale, spiral-shaped germ. Though the disease has been ravaging Europe and America for centuries, the germ of it has been discovered only a few years ago, namely, in 1905, and, like the gonococcus, also by a German scientist, Fritz Schaudinn. Syphilis is a constitutional disease. In ten days to three weeks after a person has contracted syphilis, he (or she) develops a sore (at the spot where the germs got in). This sore is called *chancre* or *primary lesion.* But when this sore makes its appearance the spirochetæ and the poison which they elaborate are already circulating in the blood, all over the system. The disease is already systemic, or constitutional, and the chancre is the local expression of a constitutional disease. Cutting out the chancre will not cure the disease, because, as stated, the germs are already in the system. The time between the contraction of the disease (the infectious intercourse) and the appearance of the chancre is called the *Incubation Period.* The time between the appearance of the chancre and the appearance of the rash on the body (the rash looks like a measles rash and is called roseola, which means a rose-colored rash) is called the *Primary Stage.* It lasts about six weeks. With the appearance of the rash commences the *Secondary Stage.* This stage is characterized by all sorts of *eruptions*, mild and severe, by white little patches (called mucous patches) in the throat, mouth, tonsils, vagina, by falling out of the hair, etc. The length of this secondary stage depends a good deal upon the sort of treatment the patient gets. Improperly treated, or not treated at all, it may last two or three years or more. Properly treated, it may be cut short at once, in a few days, so that the patient may never again in his or her life get an eruption.

The third or *Tertiary Stage* is characterized by *ulcerations* in various parts of the body and by *swellings* or tumors. The name of a syphilitic swelling or tumor is gumma (plural, gummata). The tertiary stage is the most terrible stage and it used to be the terror of syphilitic patients. But at the present time, under our modern methods of treatment, patients, if properly treated, *never have a tertiary stage.* We have seen many patients who considered syphilis a trifling disease, because all they knew of their disease was the chancre and the first eruption, i.e., the roseola, and perhaps a slight falling out of the hair. They then put themselves under energetic treatment, the *activity* of the disease was checked, and they never had another symptom afterwards, though a Wassermann test showed that the disease was not entirely eradicated. It was merely held in check—which is the second best thing.

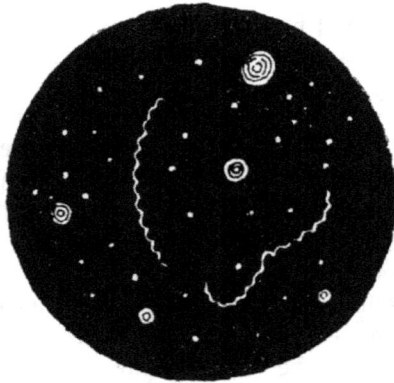

Spirocheta Pallida, or Treponema Pallidum, the Germ of Syphilis as Seen under the Microscope.

As stated before, syphilis is the most hereditary of all diseases. Fortunately, if the disease is still very active in the parents, particularly in the mother, the child is generally aborted. Some syphilitic mothers will have half a dozen or more miscarriages in succession. When the disease has become "attenuated," either by treatment or by itself—many diseases lose their virulence in time— the child may be carried to term. It then may be born dead, or it may be born strongly syphilitic, and die in a few days or weeks, or it may be born without any signs of syphilis and be apparently healthy and then develop the disease at the age of ten, twelve, fourteen, or later, or it may be born healthy and remain healthy. But no woman who had syphilis, or whose husband had syphilis, should *dare* to conceive or to give birth to a child unless she has been given permission by a competent physician. I mean just what I say. It is not a personal matter. A woman has a right to marry a syphilitic husband if she wants to and run the risk of contracting syphilis. Her body is her own, and if she does it with her eyes open it is her affair. But a woman has no right to bring into the world syphilitic or syphilitically tainted children. Here society has a right to interfere.

Syphilis runs a milder course in women than it does in men. But this milder course is not an unmixed blessing; it may be considered a misfortune, because, the same as gonorrhea in women, syphilis is often present for months and years until it has made such inroads that it is but little amenable to treatment. In many women the disease runs such a mild course, as far as definite symptoms are concerned, that they are sure they never had anything the matter with them, and they are perfectly sincere in their denial of ever having had any infection. Often it is only when they complain of obscure symptoms, for which we can find no explanation, and then take a Wassermann test, that we discover what the real trouble is. And then the internal organs are sometimes found so deeply affected that it is hard to do anything. So it is seen that the mildness of the course of the disease, while a good thing in itself, is bad in that respect that it prevents timely treatment. It is therefore important that whenever a woman is in any way suspicious that she may have the disease that she have herself examined; and if she has reasons to suspect that her husband or partner has the disease, she should persuade him to have himself examined.

Locomotor ataxia, one of the most terrible sequelæ of syphilis, is much more rare in women than it is in men. So is general paresis, also called general paralysis of the insane, or softening of the brain.

CHANCROIDS

There is one other minor disease belonging to the venereal diseases; that is chancroids. Chancroids are little ulcers on the genitals; they are purely local and do not affect the system. They are due largely to uncleanliness, and are found only among the poorer classes of prostitutes and therefore among the poorer classes of men. One sees them now and then in public dispensaries, but in private practice they are now quite rare. They used to be quite common, which shows that the general level of cleanliness has been raised considerably among all classes of people. At any rate, chancroids are of little significance, as compared with syphilis and gonorrhea, and when speaking of the venereal peril, these are the two diseases we have in mind.

CHAPTER XXVI

THE CURABILITY OF VENEREAL DISEASE

Gonorrhea May Be Practically Cured in Every Case in Man—Extensive Gonorrheal Infection in Woman Difficult to Cure—Positive Cure in Syphilis Impossible to Guarantee.

Just as the usual statements in regard to the extent of venereal disease have been found untrue or greatly exaggerated, so do the statements regarding the curability or rather incurability of venereal disease need careful revision. The picture usually painted of the hopelessness of gonorrhea and syphilis is too sombre, too black, and, contrary to the assertions made by laymen and laywomen and physicians who do not specialize in the treatment of venereal disease, I wish to make the statement that every case of gonorrhea in man, without any exception, if properly treated, can be perfectly cured, *as far as practical purposes are concerned.* I add the last phrase because the cure may not be perfect in the scientific sense of the word; that is, the man may not be brought back into the condition in which he was before he got the disease. But, for all practical purposes, as far as he himself is concerned, as far as his wife is concerned, and as far as the future children are concerned, every case may be cured, without any doubt. And I say this, basing myself upon a varied professional experience extending over nearly a quarter of a century.

As to gonorrhea in women, that depends to a great extent upon the virulence of the disease and the promptness with which treatment is instituted. If the gonorrhea is limited only to the cervix, the vulva and the urethra, then prompt treatment will usually bring about a cure in a comparatively short time. But if the gonorrheal inflammation has extended to the body of the uterus, or still worse, to the tubes, then the treatment may become a very tedious one, and some cases may not be curable without an operation.

With syphilis the matter is different. Since the introduction by Ehrlich of the various arsenic preparations, we have much better success in the treatment of syphilis, and we can positively render every case non-infectious to the partner. But, as to guaranteeing a positive cure, that is, guaranteeing that the patient will never have an outbreak or relapse of his disease in the future, and that the children will be perfectly free from any taint, this we can do no more now than we could before the modern treatment of syphilis was introduced. The decision, therefore, as to whether we may or may not permit a once syphilitic patient to marry will depend a great deal upon whether or no the husband or the wife or both desire to have children. If this is the case, we must often withhold our permission; but if the man and woman agree to get married and to get along without children, we will grant permission to the marriage in the vast majority of cases. The subject of venereal disease and marriage will be further discussed in separate chapters.

Venereal disease, I have to repeat, is terrible enough in itself, without any exaggeration, without picturing it in too black colors. And it is necessary that people should not have too black an idea of it. It is necessary that they know that there are thousands and tens of thousands of patients who suffered with gonorrhea or syphilis and who were perfectly cured, who married, and whose wives remained perfectly well, and who gave birth to perfectly healthy untainted children.

CHAPTER XXVII

VENEREAL PROPHYLAXIS

Necessity for Douching Before and After Suspicious Intercourse—Formulæ for Douches—Precautions Against Non-venereal Sources of Infection—Syphilis Transmitted by Dentist's Instruments—Manicurists and Syphilis—Promiscuous Kissing a Source of Syphilitic Infection.

In his book, *Sex Knowledge for Men,* the author treated the subject of prevention of venereal disease very thoroughly. Men need this knowledge. As men *will* indulge in illicit relations, we must teach them to guard themselves against venereal infection. We must do it not only for their own sake, but for the sake of their wives and children. For, infection in the man may mean infection in his wife and children. But as women readers of this book are not likely to indulge in promiscuous relations with strangers, a detailed discussion of the subject would be out of place.

I will merely say, that where the woman has a suspicion that her husband is in an infectious state, she should abstain from relations with him until she is sure that he is safe. But where for some reason a suspicions intercourse is indulged in, the woman should use an antiseptic douche *before* and *after* intercourse. Where it is inconvenient to use a douche both before and after, a douche after will have to suffice, but it is much safer and surer to use the douche both before and after. When you use a douche there is always some of the solution left in the vagina and that destroys wholly or in part the infective germs. The following makes an effective douche: Dissolve a tablet of bichloride (they come on the market of the weight of about 7½ grains) in two quarts of water—hot, lukewarm or cold. Use before intercourse a small amount—about a pint or half a pint, and use the balance after intercourse. Instead of the bichloride you may use a tablespoonful of carbolic acid, or two tablets of chinosol, or a tablespoonful of lysol, or two tablespoonfuls of boric acid.

Instead of the douche an antiseptic jelly in a collapsible tin tube with a long nozzle may be used.

But besides the venereal sources of infection the woman must guard against the non-venereal sources. Do not ever, if you can avoid it, use a public toilet. If you are forced to use it, protect yourself by putting some paper over the seat.

Do not use a public drinking cup. If you have to use one, keep your lips away from the rim. One can learn to drink without touching the rim of the glass or cup with the lips.

Do not under any circumstances use a public towel. The roller towel is a menace to health and should be forbidden in every part of the country.

If you have to sleep in a hotel or in a strange bed, make sure that the linen is clean and fresh. Never sleep on bed linen which has been used by a stranger.

Never use a public brush or comb.

Be sure that your dentist is a careful, up-to-date man, and sterilizes his instruments carefully. Many a case of syphilis has been transmitted by a dentist's instrument. A syphilitic who goes to a dentist to be treated generally conceals his disease, and if the dentist is not in the habit of sterilizing his instruments after each patient, disaster may result.

Be sure that your manicurist is not syphilitic, or at least that her hands are healthy, clean and free from any eruption.

And, last but not least, do not indulge in promiscuous kissing. This is a particularly important injunction for young girls. This is a real peril and there are thousands of cases of syphilis that are known to have been contracted directly from kissing. People suffering with syphilis often have little white sores (mucous patches) on their lips, tongue and inside of cheeks. These sores are very infectious, and by kissing the disease is readily transmitted. Kissing games have been responsible in more than one case for the spread of syphilis to many persons. I have now under treatment a girl of nineteen who contracted syphilis on her summer vacation from having kissed a man once. Avoid promiscuous kissing! It is a bad practice for more than one reason.

CHAPTER XXVIII

ALCOHOL, SEX AND VENEREAL DISEASE

Alcoholic Indulgence and Venereal Disease—A Champagne Dinner and Syphilis—Percentage of Cases of Venereal Infection Due to Alcohol—Artificial Stimulation of Sex Instinct in Man and in Woman—Reckless Sexual Indulgence Due to Alcohol—Alcohol as an Aid to Seduction.

That Bacchus, the god of wine, is the strongest ally of Venus, the goddess of love, using love in its physical sense, as the French use the word *amour,* has been well known to the ancient Greeks and Romans, as it is well known to-day to every saloon-keeper and every keeper of a disreputable house. And all measures to combat venereal disease and to prevent girls from making a false step will be only partially successful if we do not at the same time carry on a strong educational campaign against alcoholic indulgence. Of what use to young men is the knowledge of the venereal peril and familiarity with the use of venereal prophylactics, when under the influence of alcohol the mind is befuddled, they forget everything and do things that they never would do in the sober state? Of what use are warnings to a girl, when under the influence of a heavy dinner and a bottle of champagne, to which she is unaccustomed, her passion is aroused to a degree she has never experienced before, her will is paralyzed and she yields, though deep down in her consciousness something tells her she shouldn't? Yields, becomes pregnant, and is in the deepest agony for several months, and has a wound which will probably never heal for the rest of her life? Of what use have all the lectures, books and maternal injunctions been to her?

Or this case. Here is a young lawyer, twenty-eight years of age, engaged to a fine girl, and with everything to look forward to. He always was very moderate and circumspect in his sexual indulgence, and, though careful in choosing his partners, he never failed to use a venereal prophylactic after intercourse. There was too much at stake for him, and he did not care to take any chances, even if the chances were one in a thousand. For a period of one year during which he had been engaged he abstained from sexual intercourse altogether, though it cost him a great deal of effort to do so. He was to be married very shortly. But ill-luck made him accept an invitation to a bachelor dinner, where champagne and smutty stories were flowing freely, too freely. He left about midnight, and as the night was beautiful he decided to walk home. He met a siren, who invited him to accompany her. Under other circumstances he would have sent her on her way, or at least he would have stepped into a drugstore for a prophylactic. But, excited by the wine, the smutty stories and the year's abstinence, he went along like a sheep, as a matter of course, without trying to reason or interposing any objections. He remembers distinctly his feelings and the state of his mind. He was not drunk, only exhilarated, but nevertheless the whole thing seemed to him so normal, so natural, so expected, so matter-of-course, that he couldn't think of acting otherwise than accept her invitation. And he stayed two or three hours; and he used no prophylactic. And as a result—three weeks later he had a typical primary syphilitic lesion. How he felt and what it all meant to him the reader can imagine. This is far from being an isolated, an exceptional case.

From my own practice I could cite a number of cases of venereal infection in which alcohol was the direct, primary factor. How many such cases there are altogether in the period of a year nobody can say, but that they constitute a considerable percentage of the total venereal morbidity every investigating sexologist will testify. Forel claims that 76 per cent. of all venereal infection takes place under the influence of alcohol; Notthaft is more moderate, more discriminating in his statistics and his claims are—30 per cent. An analysis of 1,000 cases of venereal infection, just published by Dr. Hugo Hecht (*Venerische Infektion und Alkohol, Z.B.G.*, Vol. XVI, No. 11) gives over 40 per cent. And the saddest part of it is that among the infected were 75 married men (the author thinks there were more, but only 75 confessed to being married), and of these, 45, equivalent to 60 per cent., were under the influence of alcohol when they contracted their venereal disease (extra-matrimonially, of course).

Alcoholic indulgence contributes to the spread of venereal disease directly and indirectly. First and foremost it increases enormously the amount of intercourse indulged in. I certainly do not belong to those who believe that the sex instinct is merely a vicious appetite, like the appetite for alcohol or drugs, which can easily and completely be suppressed by the exertion of will-power. I believe that the sex instinct can be suppressed only within reasonable limits; if an attempt is made to exceed these limits dire results are apt to follow. But I also believe that the sex instinct can be stimulated artificially beyond the natural needs, and among the artificial stimulants of the sex instinct alcohol occupies first place. And bear in mind that alcohol produces even a stronger effect on women, in exciting the sexual passion, than it does on men. Women are more easily upset by stimulants and narcotics, and that is the reason why it is more dangerous for women to drink than it is for men.

So this, then, is count number one: The man and the woman who in a sober condition would easily abstain, with their libido stimulated and their will-power paralyzed by alcohol, indulge unnecessarily, with the risk of venereal infection to the man and the double risk of venereal infection and pregnancy to the woman. Count two: The man who in the sober condition would use care and discrimination, under the influence of alcohol soon loses all his judgment and sees an angel and a Helen of Troy in the worst and most impudent harlot; with the result that the chances of venereal infection are greatly increased. Count three: Where under ordinary circumstances the man would stay a few minutes to half an hour, under the influence of alcohol he stays several hours, or all night, thus increasing his chances of infection a hundredfold. Count four: Alcohol increases the congestion in the genital organs of both man and woman and renders them much more *susceptible* to infection. All other factors being equal, a connection which will under strict sobriety remain without bad results, may when one or both partners are under the influence of alcohol be followed by infection. Count five: The man who is in the habit of using venereal prophylactics under the influence of alcohol becomes both careless and reckless; he looks with contempt at preventive measures and the result is—venereal disease.

It is impossible to give statistics and exact or even approximate figures. But there is no question in my mind, in the mind of any careful investigator, that if alcoholic beverages could be eliminated, the number of cases of venereal infection would be diminished by about one-half. And what is true of venereal disease is also true of seduction of young girls. Alcohol is the most efficient weapon that either the refined Don Juan or the vulgar pimp has in his possession.

You cannot hope for complete success in eliminating venereal disease and seduction unless you also eliminate alcoholism. For Bacchus is the ally not only of Venus Aphrodite but also of Venus vulgivaga.

CHAPTER XXIX

MARRIAGE AND GONORRHEA

Decision of Physician Regarding Marriage of Patients Infected with Gonorrhea or Syphilis—Advisability of Certificate of Freedom from Transmissible Disease—Premarital Examination as a Universal Custom—When a Man Who Had Gonorrhea May Be Allowed to Marry—When a Woman Who Had Gonorrhea May be Allowed to Marry—Antisepsis Before Coitus—Question of Sterility in the Man Who Has Had Gonorrhea Easily Answered—Impossibility of Determining Whether the Woman is Fertile or Not.

For a man or a woman who has once suffered from gonorrhea or syphilis to enter matrimony without having secured a competent physician's opinion is a great responsibility. And a great responsibility rests upon the shoulders of the physician who is called upon to give such an opinion. For, a wrong decision—a wrong decision either way—that is, permission to marry when permission should not have been granted or refusal to give permission when permission should have been granted—may be responsible for much future unhappiness and much disease: disease of the mother and of the offspring. It may even be responsible for death.

There is no easy, short road to a positive opinion. It requires a thorough, painstaking examination at the hands of an experienced physician, one thoroughly familiar with all the modern tests, to tell whether it is safe for a man who once suffered from venereal disease to enter the bonds of matrimony. Sometimes one examination is not sufficient, and several examinations may be necessary; but, the opinion of a conscientious, experienced physician may be relied upon, and, if all men and women who once suffered from venereal disease would seek for, and be guided by, such an opinion, there would be no cases of marital infection, there would be no children afflicted with gonorrheal ophthalmia, there would be no cases of hereditary syphilis.

I firmly believe that a time will come when all venereal disease will have disappeared from the face of the earth. But, until that time comes, it would be for the benefit of the race and of posterity if people had to present a certificate of freedom from transmissible venereal disease as a prerequisite to a marriage license. Custom is often more efficient than law, and, if a premarital examination should become a universal custom (and there are indications in this direction), no law would be needed.

When May a Man Who Had Gonorrhea Get Married? For a man who once suffered from gonorrhea to be pronounced cured and a safe candidate for marriage, the following conditions must be present:

1. There must be no discharge.

2. The urine must be perfectly clear and free from shreds.

3. The secretion from the prostate gland, as obtained by prostatic massage, and from the seminal vesicles, as obtained by "milking," or "stripping," the vesicles, must be free from pus and gonococci. To make sure, it is best to repeat such examination at three different times.

4. There must be neither stricture nor patches in the urethra.

5. What we call the complement-fixation test, which is a blood test for gonorrhea similar to the Wassermann blood-test for syphilis, must be negative.

Referring to conditions 1 and 2, it sometimes happens that the patient has a minute amount of discharge or a few shreds in the urine, and I still permit him to marry; but this is done only after the discharge and shreds have been repeatedly examined and have been found to be catarrhal in character and absolutely free from any gonococci or other germs.

It sometimes happens that a patient comes to me for an examination a few days before the date set for the wedding. I examine him and find that he is not in a safe condition to marry, and so advise him to delay the wedding. Sometimes he follows the advice, but in some cases he is unable to do so. He claims the wedding has been arranged, the invitation-cards have been sent out, and to delay the wedding would lead to endless trouble and perhaps scandal. In such cases I, of course, assume no responsibility; however, I do advise the man to use an antiseptic suppository or some other method that will protect the bride from infection for the time being, while he, the husband, has an opportunity to take treatment until cured. Of the many cases in which I advised this method, I do not know of one in which infection has taken place.

When May a Woman Who Once Had Gonorrhea Be Permitted to Marry? In the case of a woman, the decision may be harder to reach than in that of a man. Of course, the urine must be clear and the urethra must be normal; however, we cannot insist that there must be no discharge. This, because practically every woman has some slight discharge; even, if not all the time, then at least immediately prior and subsequent to menstruation. Of course, the discharge must be free from gonococci and pus. Also the complement-fixation tests must be negative. But, even so, we cannot be absolutely sure, because gonococci may be hidden in the uterus or in the Fallopian tubes.

Here, we have to go a good deal by the history given us. If the woman, during the course of the gonorrhea, had salpingitis, that is, an inflammation of the Fallopian tubes, then we can never say positively that she is cured; all we can say, at best, is: presumably cured. And, further, if she has no pains in the uterine appendages, either spontaneous or on examination, and, if several examinations made within a day or two following menstruation are negative, then we may assume that she is cured. It is important, though, that this examination be made on the last day of menstruation or on the first or second day following; for there are many cases in which no pus and no gonococci will show in the inter-menstrual period, but will appear on those particular days, because, if the gonococci are hidden high up, they are likely to come down with the menstrual blood and portions of mucous membrane that are shed during menstruation.

At best, it is a delicate problem, so that whenever there has been the least suspicion that the woman may harbor gonococci I have always advised (as is my custom, to be on the safe side) and directed the woman to use either an antiseptic suppository or an antiseptic douche before coitus. With these precautions adopted, I have never had an accident happen.

The Question of Probable Sterility. Thus far I have considered the problem of marriage from the standpoint of infectivity. But, we know that, besides the effect on the individual, gonorrhea has also a far-reaching influence on the race; in other words, that it is prone to make the subjects—both men and women—sterile. And a candidate for marriage may, and often does, want to know whether, besides being noninfective, he or she is capable of begetting or having children.

In the case of man, the problem is, fortunately, a very simple one. We can easily obtain a specimen of the man's semen and determine, by means of the microscope, whether it contains spermatozoa or not. If it does contain a normal number of lively, rapidly moving spermatozoa, the man is fertile, regardless of whether he ever had epididymitis or not. If the semen contains no spermatozoa, or only a few deformed or lazily moving ones, then he is sterile.

In the case of woman, it is *absolutely* impossible to determine whether the gonorrhea has made her sterile or not; because there is no way of expressing an ovum from the ovary. The woman may not have had any pain or inflammation in the Fallopian tubes, and yet there may have been sufficient inflammation to close up the orifices of the tubes. On the other hand, she may have had a severe salpingitis on *both sides and still be fertile.* Nor is there any way of telling whether the ovaries were so involved in the process as to become incapable of generating healthy ova, or any ova at all. In short, there is absolutely no way of telling whether a woman is sterile or fertile—we can only surmise. And our surmise in this respect is liable to be wrong just as often as right. The only way the question can be decided is by experience. If the prospective husband is willing to take a chance, well and good.

While just as many girls marry as do young men, still, in practice, we always shall have to examine an incomparably larger number of male than of female candidates. This is due, not only to the fact that an incomparably larger number of men suffer from venereal disease, but also because very few women will confess to their fiancés that they ever entertained antematrimonial relations and—what is still worse—were infected with venereal disease. This, of course, is owing to our double standard of morality, which looks upon as a trivial or no offense in the man what it condemns as a heinous crime in the woman. I have known hundreds of men who confessed freely to their fiancées that they had had gonorrhea, but I have known only two girls who made a confession of the fact to their future husbands. They got married, however, and lived happily with their husbands ever after.

CHAPTER XXX

MARRIAGE AND SYPHILIS

Rules for Permitting a Syphilitic Patient to Marry—Rules More Severe in Cases Where Children Are Desired—Where Both Partners Are Syphilitic—Danger of Paresis in Some Syphilitic Patients—A Case in the Author's Practice.

The problem of the syphilitic differs from the problem of the exgonorrheal patient. When a gonorrheal patient is cured, so far as infectivity is concerned, and is not sterile, there is no apprehension as to the offspring. Gonorrhea is not hereditary, and the child of a gonorrheal patient does not differ from the child of a nongonorrheal person. In the case of syphilis, it is different. The patient may be safe so far as infecting the partner is concerned, but yet there may be danger for the offspring.

The rules for permitting a man or a woman who once had syphilis to marry, therefore, are different from those applied to the gonorrheal patient. Here are the rules:

1. I would make it an invariable rule that no syphilitic patient should marry or should be permitted to marry before *five* years have elapsed from the day of infection. But the period of time alone is not sufficient; other conditions must be met before we may give a syphilitic patient permission to marry.

2. The man or the woman must have received thorough systematic treatment for at least three years, either constantly or off and on, according to the physician's judgment.

3. For at least one year before the intended marriage, the person must have been absolutely free from any manifestations of syphilis; that is, from any eruptions on the skin, from any mucous patches, swelling in the bones, ulcerations, and so on.

4. Four Wassermann tests, taken at intervals of three months and at a time *when the patient was receiving no specific treatment,* must be absolutely negative.

If these four conditions are fully met, then the patient may be permitted to marry.

It is important, however, to state that, in permitting or refusing syphilitic persons to marry, we are guided to a great extent by the fact as to whether they *expect to have children soon or not.*

In the case of a couple who are anxious to have children soon after their marriage, the conditions for our permission must be more severe than when the couple are willing or anxious to use contraceptive measures for the first years of their married life. For, if a man is free from any skin lesions and from any mucous patches, his wife is safe from infection *as long as she does not become pregnant.* But, if she does get pregnant, she may become infected through the fetus; and, of course, the child also is liable to be syphilitic. Hence, much stricter requirements for syphilitics who expect to become parents are necessary than for those who do not.

In case both the man and the woman are or have been syphilitic, permission to marry may be granted without hesitation, as the danger of infection is absent, but permission to have children must be refused *absolutely* and *unequivocally.* Regardless of the time that may have elapsed from the period of infection, regardless of treatment, regardless of Wassermann tests, the danger to the child is too great if both parents have the syphilitic taint in them. A healthy child *may* be born from two syphilitic parents who have undergone energetic treatment, but we have no right to take the chance. I, at least, never wanted to, nor ever will want to, take such a responsibility.

The Danger of Locomotor Ataxia or Paresis. There is still one more point to consider in dealing with a syphilitic patient. In patients who did not receive energetic treatment from the very beginning of the disease as also in patients whose treatment was only desultory and irregular, we never can guarantee, in spite of lack of external symptoms, in spite of a negative Wassermann reaction, that some trouble may not develop later in life.

What shall we do in such cases and what particularly shall we do if, from a general examination of the patient, we carry away the impression that, while free from the danger of infection, the man is not a good risk? Under these circumstances, we must refuse all personal responsibility, leaving the assumption of the responsibility to the prospective wife.

Here is a case in point. About five years ago a man came to me for examination; he came with his fiancée. He had contracted syphilis ten years previously, received irregular treatment by mouth, off and on. For five years, he had had no symptoms of any kind. He *considered* himself cured, but wanted to know, and his fiancée wanted to know, whether he really was cured. There were no symptoms of any kind and the Wassermann test was negative. Nevertheless, I could not give him a clean bill of health. I noticed what seemed to me a slowness in thinking and just the least bit of hesitation in his speech.

I told the girl (the man was thirty-five, she was thirty-two) that I could not render a definite decision in the matter, that everything might be all right, and then again it might not; but, that the question about children she would have to decide definitely, once for all, namely, that she was not to have any children. She was fully satisfied so far as that part was concerned; she said she herself objected to children and did not intend to have any and knew how to take care of herself. All she wanted to know was, whether she was in danger of being infected. I told her no, but that in my opinion there was some danger of her husband developing general paresis or locomotor ataxia.

The girl had been a teacher for about twelve years, and she was so sick at heart of the work, was so anxious for a home of her own, that she decided to take the risk. And they got married. The marriage remained childless. The man developed general paresis (softening of the brain) three years later and died about a year afterward. The woman, now a widow, I understand, is not sorry for the step she had taken. This shows what things our social-economic conditions and our moral code are responsible for.

CHAPTER XXXI

WHO MAY AND WHO MAY NOT MARRY

The Physician Often Consulted as to Advisability of Marriage—*Venereal Disease* the Most Common Question—*Tuberculosis*—Sexual Appetite of Tubercular Patients—Effect of Pregnancy Contraceptive Knowledge for Tubercular Wife—*Heart Disease*—Serious Bar to Marriage—Influence of Sexual Intercourse—*Cancer*—Fear of Hereditary Transmission—*Exophthalmic Goiter*—Most Frequent in Women—Simple Goiter—Exceptions to Rule—*Obesity*—Family History—Obesity and Stoutness Not Synonymous—*Arteriosclerosis*—Danger in Sexual Act—*Gout*—Real Causes of Gout—*Mumps*—Parotid Glands and Sex Organs—Mumps and Sterility—Oöphoritis Due to Mumps—*Hemophilia*—Hemophilic Sons May Marry—Hemophilic Daughters May Not Marry—*Anemia*—*Chlorosis*—*Epilepsy*—Hysteria—Symptoms of Hysteria—Marriage of Hysterical Women—*Alcoholism*—Effect on Offspring—Alcoholics and Impotence—*Feeblemindedness*—Evil Effects on Offspring—Sterilization of Feebleminded Only Preventive—*Insanity*—Functional Insanity—Organic Insanity—Hereditary Transmissibility of Insanity—Fear Resulting in Insanity—Environment versus Heredity in Insanity—*Neurosis*—*Neurasthenia*—*Psychasthenia*—*Neuropathy*—*Psychopathy*—Nervous Conditions and Genius—Sexual Impotence and Genius—*Drug Addiction*—External Causes—*Consanguineous Marriages*—When Consanguineous Marriages are Advisable—Offspring of Consanguineous Marriages—Homosexuality—Homosexuals Often Ignorant of Their Condition—Sexual Repression and Homosexuality—Sadism and Divorce—Masochism—Sexual Impotence and Marriage—Effect Upon the Wife—Frigidity—Marital Relations and Frigid Woman—Excessive Libido and Marriage—Excessive Demands Upon Wife—Satyriasis—The Excessively Libidinous Wife—Nymphomania—Treatment—Harelip—Myopia—Astigmatism—Premature Baldness—Criminality—Crime as Result of Environment—Legal and Moral Crime—Ancestral Criminality and Marriage—Rules of Heredity—Pauperism—Difference Between Pauperism and Poverty.

In former years, nobody thought of asking a physician for permission to get married. He was not consulted in the matter at all. The parents would investigate the young man's social standing, his ability to make a living, his habits perhaps, whether he was a drinking man or not, but to ask the physician's expert advice—why, as said, nobody thought of it. And how much sorrow and unhappiness, how many tragedies the doctor could have averted, if he had been asked in time! Fortunately, in the last few years, a great change has taken place in this respect. It is now a very common occurrence for the intelligent layman and laywoman, imbued with a sense of responsibility for the welfare of their presumptive future offspring and actuated, perhaps, also by some fear of infection, to consult a physician as to the advisability of the marriage, leaving it to him to make the decision and they abiding by that decision.

As a matter of fact, as often is the case, the pendulum now is in danger of swinging to the other extreme; for, a little knowledge is a dangerous thing, and the tendency of the layman is to exaggerate matters and to take things in an absolute instead of in a relative manner. As a result, many laymen and laywomen nowadays insist upon a thorough examination of their own person and the person of their future partner, when there is nothing the matter with either. Still, this is a minor evil, and it is better to be too careful than not careful enough.

I am frequently consulted as to the advisability or nonadvisability of a certain marriage taking place. I, therefore, thought it desirable to discuss in a separate chapter the various factors, physical and mental, personal and ancestral, likely to exert an influence upon the marital partner and on the expected offspring, and to state as briefly as possible and so far as our present state of knowledge permits which factors may be considered eugenic, or favorable to the offspring, and dysgenic, or unfavorable to the offspring.

The questions concerning the advisability of marriage which the layman as well as the physician have most often to deal with are questions concerning venereal disease. On account of the importance of the subject, these have been discussed rather in detail under the headings "Gonorrhea and Marriage" and "Syphilis and Marriage." Other factors affecting marriage, either in the eugenic or dysgenic sense, will be discussed more briefly in the present chapter, and more or less in the order of their importance.

TUBERCULOSIS

Tuberculosis, which carries off such a large part of humanity every year, is caused by the well-known bacillus tuberculosis, discovered by Koch. The germ is generally inhaled through the respiratory tract, and most frequently settles in the lungs, giving rise to what is known as pulmonary consumption. However, many other organs and tissues may be affected by tuberculosis.

Tuberculosis used to be considered the hereditary disease *par excellence*. Entire families were carried off by it, and, seeing a tuberculous father or mother and then tuberculous children, it was assumed that the infection had been transmitted to the children by heredity. As a matter of fact, the disease was spread by infection. In former years, little care was exercised about destroying the sputum; the patients would spit indiscriminately on the floor, and the sputum, drying up, would be mixed with the dust and inhaled. Often the children crawling on the floor would introduce the infective material directly, by putting their little fingers in their mouths.

It is now known that tuberculosis is not a hereditary disease, that is, that the germs are not transmitted by heredity. *The weak constitution*, however, which favors the development of tuberculosis, is inherited. And children of tuberculous parents, therefore, must not only be guarded against infection, but must be brought up with special care, so as to strengthen their resistance and overcome the weakened constitution which they inherited.

That a person with an active tuberculous lesion should not get married goes without saying. But, it is a good rule to follow for a tuberculous person not to marry for two or three years, until all tuberculous lesions have been declared healed by a competent physician. As a rule, a tuberculous patient is a poor provider, and that also counts in the advice against marriage. Then sexual intercourse has, as a rule, a strong influence on the development of the disease. Unfortunately the sexual appetite of tuberculous patients is not diminished, but, rather, very frequently heightened; and frequent sexual relations weaken them and hasten the progress of the disease.

As to pregnancy, that has an extremely pernicious effect on the course of tuberculosis, and no tuberculous woman should ever marry. If such a one does marry or if the disease develops after her getting married, means should be given her to prevent her from having children. During the pregnancy, the disease may not seem to be making any progress—occasionally the patient may even seem to improve—but after childbirth the disease makes very rapid strides and the patient may quickly succumb. In the early days of my practice I saw a number of such cases. If precautions are taken against pregnancy, then permission to indulge in sexual relations may be given, provided it is done rarely and moderately.

If a patient who has tuberculosis conceals the fact from the future partner, a fraud is committed, and the marriage is morally annullable. It has been declared legally annullable by a recent decision of a New York judge.

HEART DISEASE

Heart disease also is no longer considered hereditary. Nevertheless, heart disease, if at all serious, is a contraindication to marriage. First, because the patient's life may be cut off at any time. Second, sexual intercourse is injurious for people having heart disease; it may aggravate the disease or even cause sudden death. It is more injurious even than it is in tuberculosis. Third—and this concerns the woman only—pregnancy has a *very* detrimental effect upon a diseased heart. A heart that, with proper care, might be able to do its work for years, often is suddenly snapped by the extra work put upon it by pregnancy and childbirth. Sometimes a woman with a diseased heart will keep up to the last minute of the delivery of the child and then suddenly will gasp and expire. In the first year of my practice I saw such a case, and I never have wanted to see another. Women suffering from heart disease of any serious character should not, under any circumstance, be permitted to become pregnant.

CANCER

No man will knowingly marry a woman, and no woman will marry a man, afflicted with cancer. However, this question often comes up in cases where the matrimonial candidates are free from cancer, but where there has been cancer in the family.

Cancer is not a hereditary disease, contrary to the opinions that have prevailed, and, if the matrimonial candidate otherwise is healthy, no hesitation need be felt on the score of heredity. The fear of hereditary transmission of the disease has caused a great deal of mischief and unnecessary anxiety to people. Scientifically conducted investigations and carefully prepared statistics have shown that many diseases formerly considered hereditary are not hereditary in the least degree.

Should it, however, be shown that in one family there were *many* members who died of cancer, it would indicate that there is some disease or dyscrasia in that family, and the contracting of a marriage with any member of that family would be inadvisable.

EXOPHTHALMIC GOITER (BASEDOW'S DISEASE)

Exophthalmic goiter is a disease characterised by enlargement of the thyroid gland, protrusion of the eyeballs, and rapid beating of the heart. The disease is confined almost entirely, though not exclusively, to women, and I should not advise any exophthalmic woman to marry; neither should I advise a man to marry an exophthalmic goiter woman. It is a very annoying disease, while sexual intercourse aggravates all the symptoms, particularly the palpitation of the heart. The children, if not affected by exophthalmic goiter, are liable to be very neurotic.

Simple goiter, that is, enlargement of the thyroid gland (chiefly occurring in certain high mountainous localities, such as Switzerland), is not so strongly dysgenic as is exophthalmic goiter. Still, goiter patients are not good matrimonial risks.

Of course, there are always exceptions. I know an exophthalmic goiter woman who brought up four children, and very good, healthy children they are. But in writing we can only speak of the average and not of exceptions.

OBESITY

Obesity, or excessive stoutness, is an undue development of fat throughout the body. That it is hereditary, that it runs in families, there is no question whatsoever. And, while with great care as to the diet and by proper exercise, obesity may, as a rule, be avoided in those predisposed, it none the less often will develop in spite of all measures taken against it. Some very obese people eat only one-half or less of what many thin people do; but in the former, everything seems to run to fat.

Obesity must be considered a dysgenic factor. The obese are subject to heart disease, asthma, apoplexy, gallstones, gout, diabetes, constipation; they withstand pneumonia and acute infectious diseases poorly, and they are bad risks when they have to undergo major surgical operations. They also, as a rule, are readily fatigued by physical and mental work. (As to the latter, there are remarkable exceptions. Some very obese people can turn out a great amount of work, and are almost indefatigable in their constant activity.) Each case should be considered individually, and with reference to the respective family history. If the obese person comes from a healthy, long lived family and shows no circulatory disturbances, no strong objections can be raised to him or to her. But, as a general proposition, it must be laid down that obesity is a dysgenic factor.

But bear in mind that obesity and stoutness are not synonymous terms.

ARTERIOSCLEROSIS

Arteriosclerosis means hardening of the arteries. All men over fifty are beginning to develop some degree of arteriosclerosis; but, if the process is very gradual, it may be considered normal and is not a danger to life; when, however, it develops rapidly and the blood pressure is of a high degree, there is danger of apoplexy. Consequently, arteriosclerosis and high blood pressure must be considered decided bars to marriage.

It must be borne in mind that the sexual act is, in itself, a danger to arteriosclerotics and people with high blood pressure, because it may bring about rupture of a blood-vessel. There are many cases of sudden death from this cause of which the public naturally never learns. Married persons who find that they have arteriosclerosis or high blood pressure should abstain from sexual relations altogether or indulge only at rare intervals and moderately.

GOUT

A consideration of gout in connection with the question of heredity will show how near-sighted people can be, how they can go on believing a certain thing for centuries without analyzing, until somebody suddenly shows them the absurdity of the thing. Gout was always considered a typical hereditary disease; for it was seen in the grandfathers, fathers, children, grandchildren, and so on. So, certainly, it must be hereditary! It did not come to our doctors' minds to think that perhaps, after all, it was not heredity that was to blame, but simply that *the same conditions* that produced gout in the ancestors likewise produced it in their descendants.

We know now that gout is caused by excessive eating, excessive drinking, lack of exercise, and faulty elimination. And, since, as a general thing, children lead the same lives that their fathers did, they are likely to develop the same diseases as their fathers did. A poor man who leads an abstemious life doesn't develop gout, and if his children lead the same abstemious lives they do not develop gout. (There are some cases of gout among the poor, but they are very rare.) But if they should begin to gorge and live an improper life they would be prone to develop the disease.

The disease, therefore, cannot in any way be considered hereditary. In matrimony, gout in either of the couple is not a desirable quality, but it is not a bar to marriage; and, if the candidate individually is healthy and free from gout, the fact that there was gout in the ancestry should play no rôle.

MUMPS

Mumps is the common name for what is technically called parotitis (or parotiditis). Parotitis is an inflammation of the parotid glands. The parotid glands are situated, one on each side, immediately in front and below the external ear, and they are between one-half and one ounce in weight. They belong to the salivary glands; that is, they manufacture saliva, and each parotid gland has a duct through which it pours the saliva into the mouth. These ducts open opposite the second upper molar teeth.

We might be surprised to be told that these parotid glands can have anything to do with the sex organs, but there is no other remote organ that has such a close and rather mysterious relationship with the sex-glands as have the parotids. When the parotid glands, either one or both, are inflamed, the testicles or ovaries are also liable to be attacked by inflammation. The inflammation of the testicles may be so severe as to cause them to shrivel and dry up; or, even when no shrivelling, no atrophy of the testicles occurs, they may be so affected as to become incapable of producing spermatozoa. Moreover, in cases where the testicles of a mumps patient seemingly were not attacked—that is, where the patient was not aware of any inflammation, having no pain and no other symptoms—the testicles may have become incapable of generating spermatozoa.

Besides the testicles, the prostate gland, the secretion of which is necessary to the fertility of the spermatozoa, may also become affected and *atrophied.*

It is, therefore, a very common thing for men who had the mumps in their childhood to be found sterile.

As to the sexual power of mumps patients, that differs. Some patients lose their virility entirely; others remain potent, but become sterile.

The same thing happens to girls attacked by mumps. They may have a severe inflammation of the ovaries (ovaritis or oöphoritis) or the inflammation may be so mild as to escape notice. In either case, the girl when grown to womanhood may find herself sterile.

A man who never had any venereal disease, but who has had mumps, should have himself examined for sterility before he gets married. As explained in the chapter "Marriage and Gonorrhea," we can, in the case of a man, easily find out whether he is fertile or sterile. But, in the case of a woman, we can not. Time, necessarily, has to answer that question. In all cases, mumps reduces the chances of fertility, and no man or woman who once had mumps should get married without informing the respective partner of the fact. There should be no concealment before marriage. When the partners to the marriage contract know of the facts, they can then decide as to whether or not the marriage is desirable to them.

HEMOPHILIA, OR BLEEDERS' DISEASE

Hemophilia is a peculiar disease, consisting in frequent and often uncontrollable hemorrhages. The least cut or the pulling of a tooth may cause a severe or even dangerous hemorrhage. The slightest blow, squeeze or hurt will cause *ecchymoses,* or discolorations of the skin. The peculiarity of this hereditary disease is, that it attacks almost exclusively the males, but is transmitted almost exclusively through the female members. For instance, Miss A., herself *not* a bleeder, comes from a bleeder-family. She marries and has three boys and three girls; the three boys will be bleeders, the three girls will not; the three boys marry and have children; their children will *not* be bleeders; the three girls marry, and *their male* children will be bleeders.

What is the lesson? The lesson is, that boys who are bleeders may marry, because they will most likely *not* transmit the disease; but girls who come from a hemophilic family, irrespective of whether they themselves are hemophilics or not, must not marry, because most likely they *will* transmit the disease.

ANEMIA

Anemia is a poor condition of the blood. The blood may contain an insufficient number of red blood cells or an insufficient percentage of the coloring matter of the blood, that is, hemoglobin. A special kind of anemia affecting young girls is called chlorosis.

Anemia and chlorosis cannot be considered contra-indications to marriage, because they are usually amenable to treatment. In fact, some cases of anemia and chlorosis are due to the lack of normal sexual relations, and the subjects get well very soon after marriage. But it is best and safest to subject anemic patients to a course of treatment and to improve their condition before they marry.

EPILEPSY

While epilepsy—known commonly as fits or falling sickness—is not as hereditary as it was one time thought to be, its hereditary character being ascertainable in only about 5 per cent. of cases, nevertheless, it is a decidedly dysgenic agent, and marriage with an epileptic is distinctly advised against. Where both parents are epileptics, the children are almost sure to be epileptic, and such a marriage should be prohibited by law. Under no circumstances should parents who are both epileptic bring children into the world. It should be the duty of the State to instruct them in methods of preventing conception.

HYSTERIA

Hysteria is a disease the chief characteristics of which are a *lack of control* over one's emotions and acts, the *imitation* of the symptoms of various diseases, and an *exaggerated* self-consciousness. The patient may have extreme pain in the region of the head, ovaries, spine; in some parts of the skin there is extreme hypersensitiveness (hyperesthesia), so that the least touch causes great pain; in others, there is complete anesthesia—that is, absence of sensation—so that when you stick the patient with a needle she will not feel it. A very frequent symptom is a choking sensation, as if a ball came up the throat and stuck there (globus hystericus). Then there may be spasms, convulsions, retention of urine, paralysis, aphonia (loss of voice), blindness, and a lot more. There is hardly a functional or organic nervous disorder that hysteria may not simulate.

Of late years our ideas about hysteria have undergone a radical change, and we now know that most, if not all, cases of hysteria are due to a repression or non-satisfaction of the sexual instinct or to some shock of a sexual character in childhood. Only too often a girl who was very hysterical before marriage loses her hysteria as if by magic upon contracting a *satisfactory* marriage. On the other hand, a healthy girl can become quickly hysterical if she marries a man who is sexually impotent or who is disagreeable to her and incapable of satisfying her sexually.

While hysteria, in itself, is not hereditary, it, nevertheless, is a question whether a strongly hysterical woman would make a satisfactory mother. The entire family history should be investigated. If the hysteria is found to be an isolated instance in the given girl, it may be disregarded, if not extreme; but if the entire family or several members of it are neuropathic, the condition is a dysgenic one. Marriage may be contracted, provided no children are brought into the world until several years have elapsed and the mother's organization seems to have become more stable. In some cases, a child acts as a good medicine against hysteria. In short, every case must be examined individually on its merits, and the counsel of a good psychologist or psychoanalyst may prove very valuable.

ALCOHOLISM

A good deal depends upon what we understand by alcoholism. The fanatics consider a person an alcoholic who drinks a glass of beer or wine with his meals. This is nonsense. This is not alcoholism, and cannot be considered a dysgenic factor. But, where there is a distinct habit, so that the individual *must* have his alcohol daily, or if he goes on an occasional drunken "spree," marriage must be advised against. And where the man (or woman) is what we call a real drunkard, marriage not only should be advised against, but most decidedly should be prohibited by law.

Alcoholism, as a habit, is one of the worst dysgenic factors to reckon with. First, the offspring is liable to be affected, which is sufficient in itself to condemn marriage with an alcoholic. Second, the earning powers of an alcoholic are generally diminished, and are likely gradually to diminish more and more. Third, an alcoholic is irritable, quarrelsome, and is liable to do bodily injury to his wife. Fourth an alcoholic often develops sexual weakness or complete sexual impotence. Fifth, alcoholics are likely to develop extreme jealousy, which may become pathological, even to the extent of a psychosis.

If both the husband and wife are alcoholics, then marriage between them which results in children is not merely a sin, but a crime.

We do not now come across cases so often as we used to of women marrying drunkards in the hope or with the hope of reforming them. But such cases still happen. This is a very foolish procedure. Let the man reform first, let him stay reformed for two or three years, and then the woman may take the chance, if she wants to.

FEEBLEMINDEDNESS

Feeblemindedness, in all its gradations—including idiocy, imbecility, moronism, and so on—is strongly hereditary and is one of the most dysgenic factors we have to deal with. It is the most dysgenic of all factors. It is more dysgenic than insanity. Marriage with a feebleminded person not only should be advised against, but should be prohibited by law. A feebleminded man has much fewer chances for marriage than has a feebleminded woman. Feebleminded girls, even to the extent of being morons, if pretty (as they often are) have very good chances of getting married, not infrequently getting for husbands young men of good families who themselves of course are not very strong mentally, but still are far from being considered feebleminded.

There are many cases of brilliant men—more than the public has any idea of—who married pretty, shy, demure, but withal feebleminded, girls, and the result has been in the largest percentage of cases very disastrous. In many cases all the children are feebleminded, or if not feebleminded, so weak mentally that it is impossible to make them go through any college or school. All the private tutoring is often in vain. And the brilliant father's heart breaks. It must be borne in mind that feeblemindedness or weak mentality is much more difficult to detect in a woman than it is in a man. Weakmindedness in a woman often passes for "cuteness," and as among the conservatives a woman is not expected to be able to discuss current topics, her intellectual caliber is often not discovered by the blinded husband until some weeks after the marriage ceremony.

As any instruction in the use of contraceptives would be wasted on the feebleminded, the only way to guard the race against pollution with feebleminded stock is either to segregate or to sterilize them. Society could have no objection against the feebleminded marrying or indulging in sexual relations, provided it could be assured that they will not bring any feebleminded stock into the world. After the man and the woman have been sterilized there is no objection to their getting married.

Where a normal, able or brilliant husband finds out too late that his wife's mentality is of rather a low order he is certainly justified in using contraceptives; and if he is determined to have children he will be obliged to divorce his wife. Of course this applies also to the wife of a weak minded husband.

INSANITY

Insanity may be briefly defined as a disease of the mind. We will not here go into a discussion as to what constitutes real insanity, as to what is understood by insanity in the legal sense of the term, and so on, except to note that we have two divisions.

One is functional insanity. This may be temporary, or periodical, and is due to some external cause, is curable, and is not hereditary. For instance, a person may get insane from a severe shock, from trouble, from anxiety, from a severe accident (such as a shipwreck), from a sudden and total loss of his fortune, of his wife and children (by fire, earthquake, shipwreck or railroad accident). Such insanities are curable and are not transmissible. Another example is what is known as puerperal insanity. Some women during childbirth, due probably to some toxic infection, become insane. This insanity may be extreme and maniacal in character. Still, it often passes away in a few days *without leaving any trace* and may never return again, or, if it does return, it may return only during another childbirth. This kind of insanity is not transmissible.

The second division is what we call organic insanity. This expresses itself in mania and melancholy, so-called manic-depressive insanity. This is due to a degeneration of the brain-and nerve-tissue and is hereditary.

But, our entire conception as to the hereditary transmissibility of insanity has undergone a radical change. There is hardly another disease the fear of whose hereditary character is responsible for so much anguish and torture. In former years, when there was an insane uncle or aunt or grandparent that fact weighed like a veritable incubus on the entire family. Every member of the family was tortured by the secret anguish that maybe he or she would be next to be affected by this most horrible of all diseases—disease of the mind. If an ancestral member of the family became insane at a certain age, every member of that family was living in fear and trembling until several years had passed *after* that critical age, and only then would they begin to breathe freely. Indeed, many people became insane from the very fear of becoming insane. It cannot be subject to any doubt that many people do become mentally unbalanced from the fear that they will become unbalanced. Fear has a tremendous influence on the purely bodily functions, but its influence on the mental functions is incomparably greater, and a person will often get that which he fears he is going to get.

Now the hereditary character of insanity is not taken in the same absolute sense in which it was formerly. While we still consider it a dysgenic factor, yet we recognize the paramount importance of environment; and we know that by proper bringing-up, using the expression bringing-up in its broadest sense—including a proper mental and physical discipline—any hereditary taint can be counteracted. In connection with this subject, the following very recent statistics will prove of interest.

The families of 558 insane persons cared for in the London county asylums were investigated, and, according to reports received from the educational authorities, only 15 of these (less than 3 per cent) had mentally defective children. As to the time of the birth of the children, whether before or after the attack of the insanity, we find the following figures: 56 out of 573 parents had children after their first attack of insanity, and 106 children were born after the onset of insanity in the parent; while the remaining 1259 children were born before the parent became insane.

Altogether, as will be seen from a discussion of the various factors rendering marriage permissible or nonpermissible, I am inclined to consider environment a more important factor than heredity. The purely physical characteristics bear the indelible impress of heredity. But the moral and cultural characteristics, which in the modern civilized man are much more important than the physical, are almost exclusively the results of environment.

NEUROSES—NEURASTHENIA—PSYCHASTHENIA— NEUROPATHY—PSYCHOPATHY

I will not attempt either exhaustive or concise definitions of the terms named in the caption, for the simple reason that it is impossible to give satisfactory definitions of them. The conditions which these terms designate do not constitute definite disease-entities, and many different things are understood by different people when these terms are mentioned. Only brief indications of the meaning will be given.

Neurosis is a functional disease of the nervous system.

Neurasthenia is a condition of nervous exhaustion, brought about by various causes, such as overwork, worry, fright, sexual excesses, sexual abstinence, and so on. The basis of neurasthenia, however, is often or even generally a hereditary taint, a nervous weakness inherited from the parents.

Psychasthenia is a neurosis or psychoneurosis similar to neurasthenia, characterized by an exhaustion of the nervous system, also by weakness of the will, overscrupulousness, fear, and a feeling of the *unreality* of things.

Neuropathy is a disease or disorder of the nervous system. Psychopathy is a disease or disorder of the mind.

Of late years we often hear people referred to as neurotics, neurasthenics, psychasthenics, neuropaths or psychopaths. These are undoubtedly abnormal conditions, and, taken as a general thing, they are dysgenic factors.

But a dysgenic factor in an animal *is* a dysgenic factor, and that is all there is to it. There are no two sides to the question. But if anything goes to show the difference between animals and human beings, and to demonstrate why principles of eugenics, as derived from a study of animals, can never be *fully* applicable to human beings, it is these considerations which we now have under discussion. To repeat, neuroses, neurasthenia, psychasthenia, and the various forms of neuropathy and psychopathy are dysgenic factors. But people suffering from these conditions often are among *the world's greatest geniuses,* have done some of the world's greatest work, and, if we prevented or discouraged marriage among people who are somewhat "abnormal" or "queer," we should deprive the world of some of its greatest men and women. For insanity is allied to genius, and if we were to exterminate all mentally or nervously abnormal people we should at the same time exterminate some of the men and women that have made life worth living.

And what is true of mentally abnormal is also true of physically inferior people. An inferior horse or dog *is* inferior. There is no compensation for the inferiority. But a man may be physically inferior, he may be, for instance, a consumptive, but still he may have given to the world some of the sweetest and most wonderful poems. A man may be lame, or deaf, or strabismic, he may be a hunchback or a cripple and altogether physically repulsive, and yet he may be one of the world's greatest philosophers or mathematicians. A man may be sexually impotent and absolutely useless for race purposes, yet may be one of the world's greatest singers or greatest discoverers.

In short, the eugenic problem in the human is not, and never will be, as simple as it is in the animal and vegetable kingdoms. If we want to strive after healthy, normal mediocrity, then the principles of animal eugenics become applicable to the human race. If, on the other hand, we want talent, if we want genius, if we want benefactors of the human race, then we must go very slow with our eugenic applications.

DRUG ADDICTION OR NARCOTISM

Addiction to drugs, whether it be opium, morphine, heroin or cocaine, is a strongly dysgenic factor. The addiction to the drug is of itself not transmissible, but the weakened constitution or degeneracy which is generally responsible for the development of the drug addiction is inheritable.

A few cases of drug addiction are external; that is, the patient may have a good healthy constitution, no hereditary taint, and still because during some sickness he was given morphine a number of times he may have developed an addiction to the drug. But those cases are rare. And such cases, if they are cured and if the addiction is completely overcome, may marry.

But in most cases it isn't the drug addiction that causes the degeneracy; it is the degeneracy or the neuropathic or psychopathic constitution that causes the drug addiction. And such cases are bad matrimonial risks.

And it is a very risky thing for a woman to marry an addict with the idea of reforming him. As I said about the alcoholic: Let him reform first, let him stay reformed for a few years, and then the rest is not so great.

CONSANGUINEOUS MARRIAGES

Consanguinity means blood relationship, and consanguineous marriages are marriages between near blood relatives. The physician is frequently consulted as to the permissibility or danger of marriages between near relations. The question generally concerns first cousins, second cousins, uncle and niece, and nephew and aunt.

The popular idea is that consanguineous marriages are bad *per se*. The children of near relatives, such as first cousins, are apt to be defective, deaf and dumb, blind, or feebleminded, and what not. This popular idea, as so many popular ideas are, is wrong. And still there is of course, as there always is, some foundation for it. The matter, however, is quite simple.

We know that many traits, good and bad, are transmitted by heredity. And naturally when traits are possessed by both father and mother they stand a much greater chance of being transmitted to the offspring than if possessed by one of the parents alone. Now then, if a certain bad trait, such as epilepsy or insanity, is present in a family that trait is present in both cousins, and the likelihood of children from such a marriage inheriting that trait is much greater than when the parents are strangers, the taint being present in the family of only one of the parents. But if there be no hereditary taint in the cousins' family, and, still more, if the family is an intelligent one, if there are geniuses in the family, then there cannot be the slightest objection to marriage between cousins, and the children of such marriages are apt to inherit in a strong degree the talents or genius of their ancestors. In short, if the family is a bad one, one below par, then marriage between cousins or between uncle and niece should be forbidden. If the family is a good one, above par, then marriage between relatives of that family should be encouraged.

The idea that the children from consanguineous marriages are apt to be deaf and dumb has no foundation in fact. Recent statistics from various asylums in Germany, for instance, have shown that only about five per cent. of the deaf and dumb children were the offspring of consanguineous marriages. If 95 per cent, of the deaf and dumb had *non*-consanguineous parents, how could one say that even in the other five per cent, the consanguinity was the cause? If it were the other way around, then of course we could blame consanguinity. As it is, we can assume even in this five per cent, a mere coincidence, and we have no right to say that consanguinity and deaf and dumbness stand in the relation to each other of cause and effect.

It is interesting to know that among the Egyptians, Persians, and Incas of Peru close consanguineous marriages were very common. The Egyptian kings generally married their sisters. This was common custom and if the children born of such unions were defectives or monstrosities the fact would have become quickly apparent and the custom would have been abolished. Evidently the offspring of very close consanguinity was normal, or even above normal, or the practice would not have been continued such a long time.

It is perhaps worth while noting that one of the world's greatest scientists, Charles Darwin, was the child of parents who were first cousins.

HOMOSEXUALITY

Homosexuality (homos—the same) is a perversion in which a person is attracted not to persons of the opposite but to persons of the same sex. Thus a homosexual man does not care for women, but is attracted to men. A homosexual woman is not attracted to men;

she only cares for women and may even loathe men. A homosexual, man or woman, has no right to marry. The wrong committed by a homosexual marrying is a double one: it is wrong to the partner, wrong to the children. The normal partner is bound to discover the abnormality, and if he (or she) does, then the married life is a very unhappy one. Even if the abnormal partner uses the utmost efforts to conceal the abnormality, he cannot afford any pleasure to the normal partner, because the sexual act committed under loathing cannot be satisfactory. The other wrong is committed on the offspring. Homosexuality is hereditary, and nobody has a right to bring homosexuals into the world, for there is no unhappier being than a homosexual. I know a homosexual woman, who, knowing her abnormality, married for the sake of a comfortable home. She has been successful in hiding from her husband her abnormality, he simply considering her frigid. But each sexual act costs her tortures. So far she has succeeded in avoiding pregnancy. I also know a highly refined and educated homosexual gentleman, who married before understanding his condition. Many homosexuals, not knowing that such a thing as homosexuality even exists, do not understand their own condition; they feel a little strange, a little puzzled, but they don't know that they ought not to marry. Soon after marrying his condition became clear to him, but in the meantime his wife conceived, and he is now the father of a healthy, good-looking boy. It is possible that with proper bringing up the development of any homosexual traits will be prevented. It should be borne in mind that long sexual repression is favorable to the development of homosexuality.

But to emphasize: homosexuality is a dysgenic factor, and no homosexual should marry.

SADISM

Sadism is a sexual perversion in which the person derives pleasure only when beating, biting, striking, or otherwise inflicting pain on the person of the opposite sex. The degree of cruelty varies, but all sadists should be shunned. Unfortunately the fact that a man is a sadist is often not found out until after marriage, but as soon as the wife has found it out she should leave the man and demand a divorce. Sadism is a sufficient ground for a separation or divorce.

No person with any moral feeling in him or her should be responsible for bringing children into the world with a possible sadistic heredity.

Sadistic cruelty is often of the gross, brutal, repulsive kind, but sometimes the sadist inflicts on his "beloved" object refined tortures of which only a cunning "demon" is capable. The sufferings which the wives of some sadists have to undergo are known only to themselves and to a few—very few—physicians.

MASOCHISM

Masochism is a sexual perversion in which the person, man or woman, *likes* to suffer pain, beatings, insults and other cruelties at the hands of the beloved object. It is a dysgenic factor but much less important than sadism.

SEXUAL IMPOTENCE

Sexual impotence is not hereditary, but impotence in the male either so complete that he cannot perform the act or consisting only in premature ejaculations (relative impotence or sexual insufficiency) should constitute a bar to marriage. This impotence may not interfere with impregnation; the wife may have children and the children will not be in any way defective, but the wife herself, unless she is completely frigid, will suffer the tortures of hell, and may quickly become a sexual neurasthenic, a nervous wreck, or she may even develop a psychosis. Any man suffering with impotence should have himself treated before marriage until he is cured; if his impotence is incurable, then for his own sake and for the sake of the girl or woman he is supposed to love he should give up the idea of marriage. The only permissible exception is in cases in which the prospective wife knows the nature of her prospective husband's trouble, and claims that she does not care for gross sexual relations and therefore does not mind the impotence. In case the wife is absolutely *frigid*, the marriage may turn out satisfactory. But I would always have my misgivings, and should the wife's apparently absent but in reality only dormant libido suddenly awaken there would be trouble for both husband and wife. It is therefore necessary to emphasize: in all cases of impotence—caution!

FRIGIDITY

Frigidity, as we have explained in a previous chapter, is a term applied to lack of sexual desire or sexual enjoyment in women. Of course many women before marriage are themselves ignorant of their sexual condition. Having learned to restrain their impulses, to repress any sexual stir, they themselves are often unable to say whether they have a strong or weak libido, or any at all. And whether or no a given woman would derive any pleasure from the sexual act can only be found out after marriage. Many girls, however, know very well whether they are "passionate" or not, but they wouldn't tell. They are afraid to confess to a complete lack of passion—they fear they might lose a husband.

Frigidity as an agent in marriage may be considered from two points of view: the offspring and the husband. The offspring is not affected by the mother's frigidity. A very frigid woman, if the frigidity is not due to serious organic causes, may have very healthy children and make an excellent mother. As far as the husband is concerned, it will depend a good deal on the degree of frigidity. If the woman is merely cold, and, while herself not enjoying the act, raises no objection to it, then it cannot be considered a bar to marriage. In fact many men, themselves not overstrong sexually, are praying for somewhat frigid wives. (It must be stated, however, that to some husbands relations with frigid and non-participating wives are extremely distasteful.) But when the frigidity is of such a degree that it amounts to a strong physical aversion to the act, it should be considered a bar to marriage. Such frigidity is often the cause of a disrupted home, often leads to divorce and is legally considered a sufficient cause for divorce or for the annulment of marriage, the same as impotence in the man is.

EXCESSIVE LIBIDO IN MEN

We have seen that sexual impotence is a dysgenic factor and if complete and incurable should constitute a barrier to marriage. The opposite condition is that of excessive libido. Libido is the desire for the opposite sex. A proper amount of libido is normal and desirable. A lack of libido is abnormal. And an excess of libido is also abnormal. But a good many men are possessed of an excess of libido; it is either congenital or *acquired*. Some men torture their wives "to death," not literally but figuratively. Harboring the prevailing idea that a wife has no rights in this respect, that her body is not her own, that she must always hold herself ready to satisfy his abnormal desires, such a husband exercises his marital rights without consideration for the physical condition or the mental feelings of his partner. Some husbands demand that their wives satisfy them *daily* from one to five or more times a day. Some wives who happen to be possessed of an equally strong libido do not mind these excessive demands (though in time they are almost sure to feel the evil effects), but if the wife possesses only a moderate amount of sexuality and if she is too weak in body and in will-power to resist her lord and master's demands, her health is often ruined and she becomes a wreck. (Complete abstinence and excessive indulgence often have the same evil end-results.) Some men "kill" four or five women before the fury of their libido is at last moderated. Of course, it is hard to find out a man's libido beforehand. But if a delicate girl or a woman of moderate sexuality has reasons to suspect that a man is possessed of an abnormally excessive libido, she would do well to think twice before taking the often irretrievable step.

I have spoken so far of excessive libido in normal men, that is, in men who are otherwise normal, sane and can *whenever necessary* control their desires. There is a form of excessive libido in men called satyriasis, which reaches such a degree that the men are often not able to control their desires, and they will satisfy their passion even if they know that the result is sure to be a venereal infection or several years in prison. Of course, satyriasis is a dysgenic factor; those suffering with that disorder are not normal; they are on the borderland of insanity, and not only should they not be permitted to marry, but they should be confined to institutions where they can be subjected to the proper treatment.

EXCESSIVE LIBIDO IN WOMEN

Just as we have impotent and excessively libidinous men, so we have frigid and excessively libidinous women. A wife possessed of excessive libido is a terrible calamity for a husband of a normal or moderate sexuality. Many a libidinous wife has driven her husband, especially if she is young and he is old, to a premature grave. And "grave" is used in the literal, not figurative, sense of the word. It would be a good thing if a man could find out the character of his future wife's libido before marriage. Unfortunately, it is impossible. At best, it can only be guessed at. But a really excessive libido on the part of either husband or wife should constitute a valid ground for divorce. When the libido in woman is so excessive that she *cannot* control her passion, and forgetting religion, morality, modesty, custom and possible social consequences, she offers herself to every man she meets, we use the term nymphomania. It is a disease which corresponds to satyriasis in men, and what I said of satyriasis applies with equal force to nymphomania. Nymphomaniac women should not be permitted to marry or to run around loose, but should be confined to institutions in which they can be subjected to proper treatment.

HARELIP

This is a congenital defect consisting in a notch or split in the upper lip. It is due to defective development of the embryo and is as a rule found in association with cleft palate. Probably hereditary, but is not common and is not of much importance.

MYOPIA

Myopia means nearsightedness. This defect is undoubtedly hereditary to a certain degree, but it is doubtful if, other conditions being favorable, any man would give up a girl because she is myopic or vice versa. Still, if the condition is extreme, as it sometimes is, it should be taken into consideration. And where both the man and the woman are strongly myopic some hesitation should be felt in contracting a marriage. If the husband alone is myopic, then the defect may be transmitted to the sons but not to the daughters, and these daughters may in their turn transmit the defect to their sons but not to their daughters. In other words, the defect is more or less *sex-limited*.

ASTIGMATISM

This is a defect of the eye, depending upon some irregularity of the cornea or the lens, in which light rays in different meridians are not brought to the same focus. It is to a certain extent hereditary, but plays an insignificant rôle. It is an undesirable trait, but cannot be considered a dysgenic factor.

BALDNESS

Premature baldness is a decidedly inheritable trait. And so is premature grayness of the hair. But it is doubtful if any woman would permit these factors to play any rôle in her choice of a husband.

CRIMINALITY

Almost a complete change has taken place in our ideas of criminality, and there are but very few criminologists now who believe in the Lombrosian nonsense of most criminality being inherited and being accompanied by physical stigmata of degeneration. The idea that the criminal is born and not made is now held only by an insignificant number of thinkers. We know now that by far the greatest percentage of crime is the result of environment, of poverty, with all that that word implies, of bad bringing up, of bad companions. We know that the child of the criminal, properly brought up, will develop into a model citizen, and vice versa, the child of the saint, brought into the slums, might develop into a criminal.

Then we must remember that there are many crimes which are not crimes, per se, but which are merely infractions of man-made laws, or representing rebellious acts against an unjust and cruel social order. Thus, for instance, a man or a woman who defying the law, would give information about birth control, and be convicted for the offence, would be legally a criminal. Morally he or she would be a high-minded humanitarian. A man who would throw a bomb at the Russian Czar or at a murderous pogrom-inciting Russian Governor would be considered an assassin, and if caught would be hanged; and in making up the pedigree of such a family, a narrow-minded eugenist would be apt to say that there was criminality in that family. But as a matter of fact, that "assassin" may have belonged to the noblest-minded heroes in history.

The eugenists will therefore pay little attention to criminality in the ancestry as a dysgenic factor. As long as the matrimonial candidate himself is not a criminal, the ancestral criminality should constitute no bar to the marriage. It is not likely to show itself atavistically in the children. Altogether a good deal of nonsense has been written about atavism. And people forget that the same rules of heredity that are applied to physical conditions cannot be applied to spiritual and moral qualities, the latter being much more dependent upon environment than the former. Of course the various circumstances must be taken into consideration, and each case must be decided upon its merits. No generalizations can be permitted. The *kind* of crime must always be considered.

And, furthermore, it should be borne in mind that not only is a criminal ancestry *per se* no bar to marriage, the marriage candidate himself may be an ex-criminal, may have served time in prison, and still be a very desirable father or mother from the eugenic viewpoint. A man who in a fit of passion or during a quarrel, perhaps under the slight influence of liquor, struck or killed a man is not, therefore, a real criminal. After serving his time in prison he may never again commit the slightest antisocial act, may make a moral citizen and an ideal husband and father.

This is not a plea for the under dog. For in this case, where the future of the race is at stake, all other considerations must be put into the background. I simply plead for an intelligent consideration of the subject. Many honored citizens are worse criminals and worse fathers than many people who have served prison sentences.

PAUPERISM

It may seem strange to discuss pauperism in relation to marriage and to speak of it as a hereditary factor, but it is necessary to discuss it, because considerable ignorance prevails on the subject, it being generally confused with poverty. There is a radical difference between pauperism and poverty. People may be poor for generations and generations, even very poor, and still not be considered or classed with paupers. Pauperism generally implies a lack of physical and mental stamina, loss of *self-respect* and unconquerable laziness. Of course we know now that laziness often rests upon a physical basis, being due to imperfect working of the internal glands. But whatever the cause of the laziness may be, the fact is that it is one of the characteristics of the pauper. And while we cannot speak of pauperism being hereditary, the qualities that go to make up the pauper are transmissible. No normal woman would marry a pauper, and the woman who would marry a pauper is not amenable to any advice or to any book knowledge. But men are sometimes tempted to marry daughters of paupers if they happen to be pretty. They should consider the matter very carefully, for some of the ancestral traits may become manifest in the children.

CHAPTER XXXII

BIRTH CONTROL OR THE LIMITATION OF OFFSPRING

Knowledge of Prevention of Conception Essential—Misapprehensions Concerning Birth-control Propaganda—Modern Contraceptives Not Injurious to Health—Imperfection of Contraceptive Measures Due to Secrecy—Prevention of Conception and Abortion Radically Different—More Marriages Consummated if Birth-control Information were Legally Obtainable—Demand for Prostitution Would be Curtailed—Venereal Disease Due to Lack of Knowledge—Another Phase of the Birth-control Problem—Knowledge of Contraceptive Methods Where There Was a Taint of Insanity, and the Happy Results.

No girl, and no man for that matter, should enter the bonds of matrimony without learning the latest means of preventing conception, of regulating the number of offspring. With people who consider any attempt at regulating the number of children a sin, we have nothing to argue, though we believe that there are very few people except among the lowest dregs of society who do not use some measures of regulation. Otherwise we would see most families with ten to twenty children instead of two or three. Nor do I intend to devote this chapter to a detailed presentation of the arguments in favor of the rational regulation of offspring. It would have to be merely a repetition of the arguments that I have presented elsewhere.[8] But a few points may well be touched upon here.

In spite of the fact that the subject of birth control is much better known now than it was when we first started to propagate it, still it cannot be mentioned too often, for the misapprehensions concerning it almost keep pace with the propaganda. First, there is a foolish notion that we would try to regulate the number of children forcibly, that we would compel people to have a small number of children. Nothing could apparently be more absurd, and still many people

[8] The Limitation of Offspring by the Prevention of Conception.

sincerely believe it. Nothing is further from the truth. On the contrary, much as we are in favor of birth control, we advise limitation of offspring only to those who for various reasons, financial, hereditary or hygienic, are unable to have many children. We emphatically believe that couples who are in excellent health, who are of untainted heredity, who are fit to bring up children, and have the means to do so, should have at least half a dozen children. If they should have one dozen, they would deserve the thanks of the community. All we claim is that in such an important matter as bringing children into the world, the parents who have to carry the full burden of bringing up these children should have the right to decide. They should have the means of control. They should be able to say whether they will have two or six or one dozen children.

CONTRACEPTIVE MEASURES

And the argument that contraceptives are injurious to the health of the woman, of the man, or of both, may be curtly dismissed. It is not true of any of the modern contraceptives. But even if it were true, the amount of injury that can be done by contraceptives would be like a drop of water in comparison with the injuries resulting from excessive pregnancies and childbirths. Some of the contraceptive measures require some trouble to use, some are unesthetic, but these are trifles and constitute a small price to pay for the privilege of being able to regulate the number of one's offspring according to one's intelligent desires.

The commonest argument now made against contraceptives is that they are not absolutely safe, that is, absolutely to be relied upon, that they will not prevent in absolutely every case. This is true; but there are three answers which render this objection invalid. First, many of the cases of failure are to be ascribed not to the contraceptives themselves, but to their improper, careless and unintelligent use. The best methods in the world will fail if used improperly. Second, if the measures are efficient in 98 or 99 per cent, and fail in one or two per cent., then they are a blessing. Some women would be the happiest women in the world if they could render 98 per cent. of their conjugal relations unfruitful. Third, the imperfections of our contraceptive measures are due to the secrecy with which the entire subject must necessarily be surrounded. If the subject of birth control could be fully discussed in medical books there is no doubt that in a short time we would have measures that would be absolutely certain and would leave nothing to be desired. But even such as they are, the measures are better than none, and as said in the beginning of this chapter, it is the duty of every young woman to acquire as one of the items of her sex education the knowledge of how to avoid too frequent pregnancies. In fact, I consider this the most important item in a woman's sex education, and if she has learned nothing else she should learn this. For this information is *absolutely* necessary to her future health and happiness.

A FEW EVERYDAY CASES

In my twenty years' work for the cause of rational birth control I have come in contact with thousands and thousands of cases which demonstrate in the most convincing manner possible the tragic results of forced or undesired motherhood, and of the fear of forced or undesired motherhood.

Some of the cases were in my own practice, some were related to me by brother physicians, some were described to me by the victims living in all parts of this vast country. Were I to collect and report all the cases that came to my notice during those twenty years, they would without exaggeration make a volume the size of the latest edition of the Standard Dictionary, printed in the same small type. Some of them are positively heartbreaking. They make you sick at the stupidity of the human race, at the stupidity and brutality of the lawgivers. But I do not wish to appeal to your emotions. I do not wish to take extreme and unique cases. I will therefore briefly relate a few everyday cases, which will demonstrate to you the beneficence of contraceptive knowledge and the tragedy and misery caused by the lack of such knowledge.

Case 1. This class of case is so common that I almost feel like apologizing for referring to it. She, whom I will call by the forbearing name of Mrs. Smith, had been married a little over nine years, and had given birth to five children. She was an excellent mother, nursed them herself, took good care of them, and all the five were living and healthy. But in caring for them and for the household all alone, for they could not afford a servant or a nurse-girl, all her vitality had been sapped, all her originally superb energy had dwindled down to nothing; her nerves were worn to a frazzle and she became but a shadow of her former self. And the fear of another pregnancy became an obsession with her. She dreamed of it at night, and it poisoned her waking hours in the day. She felt that she simply could not go through another pregnancy, another childbirth, with its sleepless nights and its weary toilsome days. She asked her doctor who brought her children into the world to give her some preventive, but he laughed the matter off. "Just be careful," was all the advice she got from him. And when in spite of being careful, she, horror of horrors, became pregnant again, she gathered up courage, went to the same doctor, and asked him to perform an abortion on her. But he was a highly respectable physician, a Christian gentleman, and he became highly indignant at her impudence in coming to him and asking him to commit "murder." Her tears and pleadings were in vain. He remained adamant.

Whether he would have remained as adamant if instead of Mrs. Smith, who could only pay twenty-five dollars for the abortion, the patient had been one of his society clientele, who could pay two hundred and fifty dollars, is a question which I will not answer in the affirmative or negative. I will leave it open. I will merely remark that in the question of abortion in certain specific cases the moral indignation of some physicians is in inverse proportion to the size of the fee expected. A doctor who will become terribly insulted when a poor woman who can only pay ten or fifteen dollars asks to be relieved of the fruit of her womb, will usually discover that the woman who can afford to pay one hundred dollars is badly in need of a curettement. Oh, no. He does not perform an abortion. He merely curets the uterus.

But to come back to Mrs. Smith. She went away from the indignant adamant doctor. But she was determined not to give birth to another child. She confided her trouble to a neighbor, who sent her to a midwife. The midwife was neither very expert, nor very clean. Mrs. Smith had to go to her two or three times. After bleeding for about ten days she developed blood poisoning, from which she died a few days later, at the early age of twenty-nine, leaving a disconsolate father, who in time to come will probably find consolation with another woman, and five motherless children, who will never find consolation. One may find a substitute for a wife, there is no substitute for a mother.

And such tragedies are of daily occurrence. May the Lord have mercy on the souls of those who are responsible for them.

Before I proceed further I wish to say that it is the terrible prevalence of the abortion evil, with its concomitant evils of infection, ill health, chronic invalidism and death, that more than any other single factor urges us in our birth control propaganda. And those who want to forbid the dissemination of any information about the prevention of conception are playing directly into the hands of the professional abortionists. They could not act any more zealously if they were in league with the latter and were paid by them. And having mentioned the subject of abortion, I wish to utter a note of warning. In our birth control propaganda, we must be very careful to keep the question of the prevention of conception and of abortion separate and apart. The stupid law puts the two in the same paragraph, some ignorant laymen and equally ignorant physicians treat the two as if they were the same thing, but we, in our speeches and our writings, must keep the two separate, we must show the people the essential difference between prevention and abortion, between refraining from creating life and destroying life already created; we must show the viciousness of meting out the same punishment for two things which are fundamentally different, different not only in degree but in kind—and it is only by thus keeping the two things apart, by showing that we stand for one thing—prevention—and not for the other—abortion, that we can ever gain the general sympathy of the public and the co-operation of the legislators. I do not say that there are not many cases in which the induction of abortion is not only justifiable, but imperative; but that is a different question, and the two issues must not be confused. And we would and should resent any attempt on the part of either enemy or friend to so confuse them.

Case 2. Mr. A. and Miss B. are in love with each other. But they cannot get married, for his salary is too small. They might risk getting married, if the specter of an indefinite number of children did not stretch out its restraining hand. She comes from a good family, she was brought up, if not in the lap of luxury, in the lap of comfort and coziness, and it is the ambition of every good American to furnish his wife at least as good a home as her father gave her. Her father, by the way, died prematurely from overwork in trying to give all possible comforts and advantages to a bevy of six unmarried and marriageable daughters.

As I said, the fear of children kept them back. Each year the hope revived that in another year their union in matrimony would be consummated. But the years passed. Mr. A.'s hair became thin and grayish, Miss B began to look haggard and pinched—and still the marriage could not take place. Miss B was very religious and very proper, and would not do anything that was improper. A was not quite so proper; he paid occasional visits elsewhere, and as instruction in venereal prophylaxis was not included in his college course, he acquired a gonorrhea, which it took him about six months to get rid of. To shorten the story, A was thirty-nine and Miss B was thirty-five when the many times postponed marriage was consummated, but Cupid seemed to be busy elsewhere when the ceremony took place, and there is very little romance in their married life. The marriage has remained childless, as I told Mr. A it would be.

I consider this a ruined life—and all for the lack of a little knowledge.

If the anti-preventionists, those who are opposed to any information about the prevention of conception, were not so hopelessly stupid, they would see that from their own point of view it would be better if such information were legally obtainable. For it would be instrumental in causing more marriages which otherwise remain unconsummated, and by favoring early marriages, it would be instrumental in curtailing the demand for prostitution, in diminishing venereal disease. And as is well known, venereal disease is one of the great factors in race suicide.

Case 3. A young woman was married to a man who besides being a brutal drunkard was subject to periodic fits of insanity. Every year or two he would be taken to the lunatic asylum for a few weeks or months, and then discharged. And every time on his discharge he would celebrate his liberty by impregnating his wife. She hated and loathed him, but could not protect herself against his "embraces."

And she had to see herself giving birth to one abnormal child after another. She begged her doctor to give her some means of prevention, but that boob claimed ignorance, and the illegality of the thing. The woman finally committed suicide, but not before she had given birth to six abnormal children, who will probably grow up drunkards, criminals or insane.

And because we object to such kind of breeding, we are accused of being enemies of the human race, of advocating race suicide, of violating the laws of God and man. Oh, for a mighty Sampson to strike the imbeciles with the jaw of an ass, for a mental Hercules to loosen the fontanelles of their petrified skulls and put some sense into them!

Case 4. This observation concerns a couple both of whom had a very bad heredity. The blood of each was badly tainted. The doctor who had treated the husband cautioned them and told them that they had no right to have children. But here the tables were turned. The doctor wanted to give them the means for prevention, but the husband and wife, pious Roman Catholics, would not go against their religion and God (as if God wanted a world full of imbeciles), and refused to employ any precautions. They have had four children so far. One of them seems fairly normal, except that he is silly, in which respect he is merely like his parents; two are deaf and blind in one eye; the fourth is a cretin, practically an idiot.

This case brings us face to face with another phase of the problem. What should we do when the parents, stupid and ignorant, refuse to stop breeding worthless material? Eugenic agitation, education, will bring about such a strong public opinion that none but idiots, who will be vasectomized or segregated, will dare to bring into the world children that are physically and mentally handicapped.

Case 5. This couple had been married eight years, and had five children And the wife said she could not stand it any more. Another child—no, she preferred death. They practiced coitus interruptus for a while, with mutual disgust, but when the wife was caught again, she said: "No more!" And she would not let her husband come near her. He could do what he pleased—she did not care. After a few months he began to go elsewhere—contracted syphilis, had to give up his position, the home was broken up, the wife went out to work, the children are scattered—in short, a home, which we are told is the foundation of our society, is broken up, and there is misery and wretchedness all around—and all for the lack of a little timely information.

Case 6. Mr. A and Miss B, twenty-eight and twenty-five years old respectively, have known one another for several years, and in spite of their occupation, which is supposed to make people blasé and cynical—he being a reporter and she a special story writer—are quite in love with each other. But their occupation and income are such that they cannot possibly afford to have and to bring up any children. They would love to get married, but the specter of a child—or rather of children—frightens them; and they remain single, to the great physical and mental injury of both. Accidentally they learn of appropriate means of regulating conception, get married and live happily—ever after, that is, until they find themselves in a position to have children and to bring them up properly.

In what way was society injured by this young couple acquiring contraceptive information?

Case 7. Mr. C and Miss D are in love with each other. Unfortunately there is a strong hereditary taint of insanity on both sides. They are too high-minded to think of giving birth to children. They might be all right, but with insanity one does not take any chances. The thing is too terrible. They are condemned to a life of celibacy, which to them means a life of loneliness and misery. But like an angel from heaven comes to them the knowledge that one can live a love-life without any penalties attached to it. They get married and there is not a happier couple living.

In what way has society been injured by this couple obtaining the contraceptive knowledge?

Case 8. Mr. and Mrs. E have been married five years. They have a child four years old which shows unmistakable symptoms of epilepsy. They are horrified and an investigation discloses the fact that on her side in the preceding generation there was a good deal of epilepsy. Of course, the next child may not be epileptic. But then again it may. No parents with any sense of responsibility would take such chances. They decide to give up conjugal relations. They keep it up for about thirteen or fourteen months; then one night an accident happens and very soon she finds herself pregnant. She declares she would rather die than to give birth to and have to take care of another epileptic child. She goes to a friendly physician who performs an abortion on her, and now the couple, not secure against future accidents, if they live together, decide to separate, and a tragedy is in sight. Fortunately they learn that conception can be prevented, and they continue to live together with benefit to themselves and harm to none.

In what way has society been injured by those people acquiring contraceptive information?

Case 9. Mr. and Mrs. F have been married six years, and in these six years they have been blessed with four children. When he married he was getting twenty-two dollars a week, and that is exactly what he is getting now. In the meantime the cost of living has gone up twenty-five per cent., and there are four extra mouths to feed and four extra bodies to clothe. What difference this has made in that little household can better be imagined than stated. The little mother has aged sixteen years in those six years, and there is not a trace left of her girlishness and youthfulness. She loves her children, and does not want to get rid of them. She would not take a million dollars for one of them, but she would not give five cents for another. But this is just what terrifies them; the possibility of another. And that possibility makes her irritable, makes her repel her husband's slightest advances, makes her move his bed to another room. She even tells him to satisfy his sexual desires elsewhere—and at the same time she is in fear and trembling that he might follow her advice. In short, a nice young home is about to be disrupted. Fortunately he reads somewhere an article on the subject of voluntary limitation of offspring, he begins to investigate; his physician pleads ignorance, but he is persistent, the physician investigates and obtains the desired information, which he shares with the patient. Harmony is restored and a happy home is re-established.

Who was injured by the couple obtaining this information? And if nobody was injured, and everybody concerned was benefited, then why should the imparting of such information be considered a felony, punishable like the most atrocious of crimes?

Case 10. Mr. and Mrs. G have been married fifteen years. They were the parents of seven children, a large enough number for any family. Those seven children were born during the first eleven years of their married life. During the past five years, afraid of having any more, they first abstained and then adopted a method which every modern sexologist knows is injurious to the nervous system of both the man and the woman. The man became a wreck; first neurasthenic, then impotent, cranky and grouchy, unable to get along in the office, constantly squabbling with his wife, who became just as bad a wreck. Their economic condition plus too many small children prevented the parents' separation. They remained living together, but they lived like a cat and a dog tied in a bag. Each silently prayed to be rid of the other. But a conversation overheard at a Turkish baths establishment put him on the right trail, and one year later we find the couple reconciled, both in good health and living a peaceful and fairly harmonious life. And those who have benefited most by the change are the children. In what way was society injured? And still if the doctor who gave Mr. G the information should have been caught and convicted, he would have been sent to prison for a year or two or five. Would he have deserved it? Here we have several plain, simple, unvarnished and unembellished cases which are typical of millions of similar cases and which prove conclusively that the law against imparting information about preventing conception is brutal, vicious, antisocial. Should not such a law be repealed, wiped off the statute books?

CHAPTER XXXIII

ADVICE TO GIRLS APPROACHING THE THRESHOLD OF WOMANHOOD

The Irresistible Attraction of the Young Girl for the Male—The Unprotected Girl's Temptations—Some Men Who Will Pester the Young Girl—Risk of Venereal Infection—Danger of Impregnation—Use of Contraceptives by the Unmarried Woman May Not Always Be Relied Upon—Nature of Men who Seduce Girls—Exceptions—Illegitimate Motherhood—Difficulties in the Way of Illegitimate Mother Who Must Earn Her Living—The Child of the Foundling Asylum—Social Attitude Towards Illegitimacy Responsible for Abortion Evil—Dangers of Abortion—The Girl Who Has Lost Her Virginity.

When a girl has passed the transition period of puberty and is entering upon young womanhood she exerts an irresistible attraction on the male sex. Whether she give the impression of a luscious red rose or of a delicate white lily, the charms of a beautiful, healthy, bright girl of seventeen or eighteen are undeniable and their appeal to the esthetic and sexual sense of every normal male is a normal, *natural* phenomenon. Whether it is a good thing or a bad thing that it is so, we will not stop to discuss here. But it is a natural phenomenon, a natural law, if you will, and one does not quarrel with natural phenomena. It is useless. But the attraction which the girl exercises on the male is fraught with danger to her, and therefore a few words of advice and of warning are not out of place.

Temptations. Fortunate are you, my young girl friend, if you come from a well-sheltered home, if you have been properly brought up, if you have a good and wise mother who knows how to take care of you. A mother's wise counsel given at the proper time, and her comradeship all the time, are more invulnerable than an armor of bronze and more secure than locked doors and barred windows. But if you have lost your mother at an early age, or if your mother is not of the right sort—it is no use hiding the fact that some mothers are not what they should be—if you have to shift for yourself, if you have to work in a shop, in an office, and particularly if you live alone and not with your parents, then temptations in the shape of men, young and old, will encounter you at every step; they will swarm about you like flies about a lump of sugar; they will stick to you like bees to a bunch of honeysuckle.

I do not want you to get the false idea that all men or most men are bad and mean, and are constantly on the lookout to ruin young girls. No. Most men are good and honorable and too conscientious to ruin a young life. But there are some men, young and old, who are devoid of any conscience, who are so egotistic that their personal pleasure is their only guide of conduct. They will pester you. Some will lyingly claim that they are in love with you; some perhaps will sincerely believe that they are in love with you, mistaking a temporary passion for the sacred feeling of love. Some will even promise to marry you—some making the promise in sincerity, others with the deliberate intent to deceive. Still others will try to convince you that chastity is an old superstition, and that there is nothing wrong in sexual relations. In short, all ways and means will be employed by those men to induce you to enter into sexual relations with them.

Don't you do it!

I am not preaching or sermonizing to you. I am not appealing to your religion or your morals. For if you have strong religious or moral ideas against illicit sexual relations, you are not in need of mine or anybody else's advice. But I assume that you are a more or less modern girl, with little or no religious bringing-up, or perhaps a radical girl, who has shaken off the shackles of religion and tradition. And to you I say: *Don't you do it.* Why? Because your welfare, your future happiness, is at stake. I am speaking from the point of view of your own good, and from that point of view I say: Resist all attempts which men make exclusively for the purpose of satisfying their sexual desire, their lust.

You will ask again, why? For several reasons. First, you run the risk of venereal infection. The danger is not so great now as in former times, but is great enough. There are still plenty of men dishonest enough to indulge in sexual relations with a woman when they know they are not radically cured. The same man who will not get married unless he is sure that he is perfectly cured will not hesitate to subject a transient girl or woman to the risk of venereal infection. I know personally, because I have treated them; yes, I treated several intelligent and radical young men who infected young girls. And some of these girls in their turn, through ignorance and innocence, infected other men. So then, the first danger is the danger of venereal infection.

The second danger, still greater and more certain than the first, is the danger of impregnation. And pregnancy for a girl under our present moral and social-economic conditions is a terrible calamity. She is ostracized everywhere, and it means, if discovered, her social death. But you will say: "Aren't there any remedies that can be used to prevent conception? Aren't you yourself among the world's chief birth-controllers; one of the world's chief advocates of the use of contraceptives?" Yes, my dear young lady, but I never made the claim that the contraceptives were *absolutely* infallible, I never claimed that they were *100 per cent.* effective in *100 per cent.* of *all* cases. But if they are effective 999 times or even 990 times in every 1000 they are a blessing. And thousands of families so consider them. And if a married woman gets caught once in a while, the misfortune is not so great. But if the accident happens to a non-married woman, the misfortune *is* great. Then again, you want to bear in mind that accidents are less likely to happen to married than to non-married women. The married woman has no fear, needs no secrecy, and she can go about the method of preparation carefully, with deliberation. The unmarried girl, *as a rule*, has not the proper conveniences, more or less secrecy must be maintained, hurry is not infrequently necessary, and that is why accidents are more apt to occur in spite of the use of contraceptives. So then, the second danger, even more sinister than the first, is the danger of pregnancy. "But if a misfortune happens, can I not have an abortion produced?" No, not always. Physicians willing to induce an abortion are not found on every corner. But this is not the principal point. What I have to say on the subject, I will say later on in this chapter.

Then it is well for you to bear in mind that those very men who use their utmost efforts, who strain every fibre and every nerve to get you, will despise you and detest you as soon as they have succeeded in making you yield to their wishes. This is one of the worst blots on the male man's character, a blot from which the female character is entirely free. And some men—fortunately their number is not very large—are such moral skunks that they take morbid pleasure in boasting publicly of their sexual conquests, and unscrupulously peddle about the name of the girl whom, by cunning false promises or other means, they succeeded in seducing. And of course such a girl finds it difficult or impossible to get married, and must end her days in solitude, without the hope of a home of her own.

For the above reasons I advise you earnestly and sincerely not to yield to the solicitations of thoughtless or unscrupulous men, who think of nothing but their coarse sensual pleasures. It is advice dictated by common sense, by your own deeper interest, aside from any religious or moral considerations.

The above advice, or call it sermon if you will, is meant principally for young girls, girls between the ages of eighteen and twenty-five. If a girl has reached the age of twenty-eight or thirty and is willing to enter upon illicit sexual relations with her eyes open, with a full knowledge of the possible consequences, then it is her affair, and nobody shall say her nay. Nobody has a right to interfere.

Nor should my advice be understood as directed to cases where there is sincere reciprocal affection and a mutual understanding. This is an entirely different matter, and has nothing to do with cases where the man is the pursuer or seducer and the woman an unwilling or reluctant victim.

But whatever the relations between the man and the girl may be, whether she yielded in a fit of passion, or was seduced by false promises, by "moral" suasion, by hypnotic influence or by the vulgar method of being made drunk, what is she to do if she finds herself, to her horror, in a pregnant condition? There are two ways open to her: either let the pregnancy go to term or to have an abortion brought on.

If she lets the pregnancy go to term she has the alternative of bringing up the child herself openly or of placing it secretly in a foundling asylum. In the first case, the necessity of publicly acknowledging illegitimate motherhood requires so much moral courage that not one woman in a thousand is equal to it. It is not moral courage alone that is required; the social ostracism could be borne with stoicism and even with equanimity, if with it were not frequently associated the fear or the real danger of starvation. For under our present system the illegitimate mother finds many avenues of activity closed to her. A school teacher would lose her position instantly, and so would a woman in any public position. It is feared that her example might have a contaminating influence on the children or on her fellow workers. Nor could she be a social worker—I know of more than one woman who lost her position with social or philanthropic institutions as soon as it was discovered that she did not live up strictly to the conventional code of sex morality. Nor could she be a private governess.

It is thus seen that to acknowledge one's self an illegitimate mother requires so much courage, so much sacrifice, that very, very few mothers are now found that are equal to the task. Especially so when it is taken into consideration that the humiliations and indignities to which the child is subjected and the later reproaches of the child itself make the mother's life a veritable hell. So this alternative is generally out of the question.

To give the child to a foundling asylum or to a "baby farm" means generally to condemn it to a slow death—and not such a slow one, either. For as statistics show about ninety to ninety-five per cent. of all babies in those institutions die within a few months. And the very few who survive and grow up have not a happy life. Life is hard enough for anybody; for children who come into the world handicapped by the disgrace of illegitimacy, life is torture indeed. It is with a breaking heart generally and because there is no other way out of the dilemma that a mother puts her baby away in a foundling asylum. She hopes and prays for its speedy death.

Taking into consideration the pitifully unhappy lot of the illegitimate mother and illegitimate child, it is no wonder that every unmarried woman, as soon as she finds herself pregnant, is frantically determined to get rid of the child in the womb as soon as possible. And abortion thrives in every civilized country. Thousands and thousands of doctors and semi-doctors and midwives are making a rich living in this country from practicing abortion. The greater the disgrace with which illegitimacy is considered in a country, the stricter the prohibition against the use of measures for the prevention of conception, the greater the number of abortions in that country. But abortion is not a trifle, to be undertaken with a light heart. It is true that if performed by a thoroughly competent physician, with all aseptic precautions, it is practically free from danger. But when performed by a careless physician or an ignorant midwife, trouble is apt to happen. Blood poisoning may set in, and the patient may be very sick for a time, and may on recovery from the acute illness remain a chronic invalid for life. And occasionally the patient dies. Whether or not abortion is justifiable under special circumstances is a separate question, which I have discussed in another place. But leaving aside the ethics of the question, if you have determined to have an abortion produced, be sure to go to a conscientious physician, and avoid the quacks and midwives. An unexpected and undesired pregnancy is punishment enough and there is no reason why you should be further punished by becoming a chronic invalid or by paying with your life. There is no sense in it. Nobody will profit by your invalidism or your death.

I do not wish to leave this topic without re-emphasizing the fact that abortion is not a trifle, to be undertaken or even to be spoken of lightly. Too many women, not only in the radical ranks, but in the conservative ranks as well, are in the habit of considering abortion as a joke, a trifling annoyance, something like a cold in the head, which, while disagreeable, is sure to pass away in a day or two. They know Mrs. A and Mrs. B and perhaps Miss C who had abortions produced on them and in two or three days they were as good as ever. Yes. But they do not know Miss D who is resting in her grave, nor do they know why Miss E and Mrs. F are invalids for life. The women who get over their abortion experiences easily are apt to talk of their good luck; the women who have become chronic invalids or who are resting in their graves as a result of an abortion are not apt to talk of the matter.

And therefore, once more, remember, an abortion is no trifling matter.

One other piece of advice and I am through. Some men of a low moral and mental caliber are under the influence of the pernicious idea that if a girl has lost her virginity—no matter under what circumstances—she no longer amounts to much and is free prey for everybody who may want her. And, like beasts of prey, these wretched specimens of humanity pester such a girl with much more impudence, more brazenness than they dare to employ in the case of a girl who is still considered a virgin. And, what is more, the girls themselves become poisoned with this pernicious idea and dare not offer the same resistance that the virgin does. And they often yield with resignation, though against their will, and though they may experience a feeling of disgust against the man.

Now again, *don't you do it.* Do not nurse the medieval idea that because you are not a virgin in the physical sense, you are "ruined," "no good," and an outcast. You are nothing of the kind. If through some cause or other you are no longer in possession of an intact hymen, it is your affair or misfortune, and nobody else's. Do not on that account cast your eyes down and avoid meeting people. Carry your head high, do not fear to meet people, and treat with contempt the jeers of the stupid and ignorant. A person's entire character does not depend upon the presence or absence of the hymen, and one misstep should not ruin a person's whole life. A boy is not "ruined," is not an outcast, because he has had sexual relations before marriage, and while the boy's and girl's cases are not exactly identical, still the poor girl should not be made to expiate one error all her life long.

It isn't fair.

CHAPTER XXXIV

ADVICE TO PARENTS OF UNFORTUNATE GIRLS

Attitude of Parents Towards Unfortunate Girl—The Case of Edith and What Her Father Did—The Pitiful Cases of Mary B. and Bridget C.

Suppose you are the parents of a girl to whom a misfortune has happened. I admit it is a misfortune, a catastrophe. Probably the greatest catastrophe that, under our present social system, can happen to an unmarried young woman. What are you going to do? Are you going to disgrace her—incidentally disgracing yourselves—are you going to kick her out of the house, condemning her to a suicide's grave, or to a life that is often worse than death? Or are you going to stand by her in her dark hours, to shield her, to surround her with a wall of protection against a cruel and wantonly inquisitive world, and thus earn her eternal gratitude, and put her on the path of self-improvement and useful social work? Which shall it be? But before you decide, kindly bear in mind that your girl is not entirely to blame; that some of the blame lies with you. If she had been *properly* brought up, this would not have happened. I know such a thing could never have happened in my household. But I know how I would have acted if such a thing had happened. And I will tell you how one father and mother did act under the circumstances.

They were far from rich; just fairly comfortable; they had a well-paying store. Edith was their treasure, because she was so pretty and so full of life. Unfortunately, she was too pretty and too full of life. She was only seventeen, but was fully developed, and had many empty-headed young admirers, who showered upon her silly compliments and cloying sweets. She became frivolous and flirtatious and was beginning to do poorly in high school. She failed in her last year, and refused to take the year over again. Now, all the time being her own, and having nobody to give any account to, she began to go out a good deal, and more than ever indulged in flirtations. One night she stayed out later than usual, her parents were worried, and when she came home about two in the morning there was a quarrel, and the father, who was a strict, impulsive man, gave her a pretty good beating. After that she went out very little, kept to herself, became rather melancholy, lost her appetite, and did not sleep well. To all inquiries she answered that there was nothing the matter with her, that she just felt a little indisposed. Four or five months thus passed.

But finally the condition could no longer be concealed. The mother was the first one to discover it. When the fact dawned upon her consciousness that her beautiful, not quite eighteen-year-old Edith was pregnant she promptly fell in a faint and it took Edith and the maid quite some time to restore her to consciousness. She became distracted. She floundered about pitifully, not knowing what to do, what decision to reach. She tried to conceal the matter from the father, but he saw that there was something wrong and it didn't take him long to worm the truth out of her. As the mother on learning the tragic truth had taken refuge in a dead faint, so he took refuge in a Berserker rage. He fumed and stormed and was in danger of an apoplectic stroke. He wanted to strike the daughter, but the mother interfered. He then ordered Edith to get out of the house and never to cross his threshold again. Edith looked at him to see if he meant it; the mother tried to intercede; but he was inflexible, and demanded that she leave at once. Edith began to gather a few of her belongings, the tears silently rolling down her face.

And here a sudden change came over the father. Some men (and women) are crushed by small misfortunes; real catastrophes awaken their finer qualities, which lay dormant within them and which might have remained dormant within them forever. In these few minutes he seems to have undergone a complete metamorphosis. He went up to Edith, took her in his arms, kissed her, told her to stay, to calm down and they would see what could be done. In a few days she was taken over to a physician who performed an abortion. She was a pretty sick girl for about six weeks, and at one time there was danger of blood poisoning setting in. But she recovered. And she was a different girl. She had shed her frivolity and lightheartedness like an old garment. She took her last year in high school over again, entered Barnard, from which she was graduated among the very first, and soon began to teach in that very high school in which she had been a pupil. One of the teachers fell in love with her and she fell in love with him. He asked her to marry him. She wanted no skeleton from the past coming down rattling its bones and marring their married life, and she told him of the unfortunate incident. A good test, by the way, to find out a man's real love and breadth of character. Fortunately the man's love was a true love, not merely passion, and he was truly broadminded, which is not a very common thing among school-teachers. Their married life is an uncloudedly happy one. And the relation between the daughter and the parents is one of sincere love and deep mutual respect.

Isn't it better so?

Didn't Edith's parents act more decently, more kindly, more humanely, more wisely than the parents, say, of Mary B, who, when they found out her condition, put her out of the house, into which she was brought back two days later a corpse, fished out from the East River? Didn't Edith's father act more nobly, more wisely even from a purely selfish point of view than the father of Bridget C, who kicked his daughter out penniless into the street, where he had to see her afterwards powdered and painted soliciting men and boys? The mother died of a broken heart, and the father, unable to bear the constant, daily repeated disgrace, became an incorrigible drunkard.

Fathers and mothers! So bring up your daughters, so guard them and protect them, that the misfortune of an illegitimate pregnancy may not befall them. But if the misfortune has befallen them, then stand by them! Do not desert them then in these dark hours, the darkest hours in a girl's life. Do not kick them—they are down enough. Stand by them, and they will become good women and you will have their eternal gratitude. If you do not stand by them, you are worse than the beasts of the jungle and deserve their eternal curse. You are unworthy to be, or to be called, parents, for you are devoid of the least spark of that sacred feeling called Parental Love, a feeling which unfortunately in only too many parents is replaced by nothing but the most sordid, most brutal egotism.

CHAPTER XXXV

SEXUAL RELATIONS DURING MENSTRUATION

Heightened Sexual Appetite of Many Women During Menstruation—Sexual Intercourse During Menstrual Period—When Intercourse May be Permitted—Injection Before Coitus During Menstruation—Fallacy of Ancient Idea of Injuriousness.

This may seem to some a strange and superfluous question, a question which would never present itself. Still the laity would be surprised if it learned how frequently nowadays that question is presented to the physician who specializes in sex matters. Some husbands come to the physician complaining that the menses are the only period during which their wives demand sex relations, and ask if something cannot be done to cure them of what they consider an abnormal desire.

Biologically considered, the desire on the woman's part for sex relations during the menses should not seem strange or abnormal, for we must bear in mind that menstruation bears a certain analogy to the rut in animals. And animals permit intercourse at no time except during the rut.

Recent investigations have disclosed to fact that the number of women whose sexual appetite is *heightened* during the time immediately preceding, during, and following the menses, is quite considerable. And there is also a smaller percentage of women who experience the desire *at no other time except* during the menses.

Speaking generally, relations during the menses should be discouraged. There are several reasons for it. The first reason, which need not be gone into in detail, is an esthetic one. The second reason is that intercourse during menstruation may in some cases lead to congestion of the uterus and ovaries. Third, the menstrual discharge, which as we know does not consist of pure blood but is a mixture of blood, mucus, and degenerated lining membrane of the uterus, may give rise to a catarrh of the urethra in the man. Fourth, and this is a point to be borne in mind, any discharge that a woman may be suffering from is always aggravated during menstruation. For these reasons relations during the menses are undesirable.

But where the woman has strong libido during that time and has no libido at any other time, relations may be indulged in during the last day or two of the menses. Any unpleasantness may be obviated and any discharge may be removed by the woman taking a mild, warm, antiseptic injection before coitus. The ancient idea of the injuriousness of the relations during menstruation and the disastrous results likely to follow them have only a very slender foundation. They rest on no scientific basis and though it may be sad to state facts, there are many couples who do indulge in such relations as a regular thing and without any injury to either husband or wife.

CHAPTER XXXVI

SEXUAL INTERCOURSE DURING PREGNANCY

Complete Abstinence During-Pregnancy—Bad Results of Complete Abstinence—Intensity of Relations During First Four Months—Intercourse During Fifth, Sixth and Seventh Months—Intercourse During Eighth and Ninth Months—Abstinence After Birth of Child.

The question whether sexual intercourse is permissible during pregnancy is often put to the physician. Some extremists and theorists demand complete abstinence during the entire duration of pregnancy. Such abstinence is not only not feasible, but is unnecessary and may prove a disrupting factor; it may create not only dissension, it may wreck the love-life of husband and wife. I know of cases where the wife, influenced by the wrong teachings about the necessity of complete abstinence during pregnancy, about the possible injury to the child from intercourse, persisted in keeping the husband away; and the result was that the husband began to go to other women, and he got in the habit to such an extent that he refused to give up entirely, even after the child was born. It cannot be expected from a married man, who is used to more or less regular sexual relations, to abstain entirely for nine or ten months. Such a demand is unreasonable and uncalled for. All claims about the injurious effects of intercourse on the mother and child lack proof and foundation. During the first four months of pregnancy no change need be made in the usual sex relations. Their "intensity" should be moderated, their frequency need not. During the fifth, sixth and seventh months intercourse should be indulged in at rarer intervals—once in two or three weeks—the act should be performed without any violence or intensity, and the usual position should be reversed or changed to a lateral one. During the eighth and ninth months relations had best be given up altogether.

And this abstinence should last until about six weeks after the birth of the child. During this period the uterus undergoes what we call involution; that is, it goes back to the size and shape it had before pregnancy, and it is best not to disturb this process by sexual excitement, which causes engorgement and congestion.

CHAPTER XXXVII

SEXUAL INTERCOURSE FOR PROPAGATION ONLY

Belief in Sexual Intercourse for Propagation Only—What Such Practice Would Lead to—Nature and the Sex-fanatics—Sexual Desire in Woman After Menopause—Sex Instinct of Sterile Men and Women—Sex Instinct Has Other High Purposes.

Some people sincerely believe that the sexual instinct is for reproductive purposes only; they claim we should never indulge in sexual intercourse unless it be for the purpose of bringing a child into the world. The act performed without such aim in view is stigmatized by them as carnal lust, as a sin. Some even say that such an act is equivalent to an act of prostitution. To *argue* the question with such people would be a waste of time. It is not fair to impugn the good faith, the sincerity of your opponents, because I have convinced myself that the most insane, most bizarre notions may be held by otherwise sane people in perfect sincerity. But we cannot help questioning the reasoning faculties of people holding such beliefs.

Let us see where the belief of "sex relations for procreation only" would lead us to. In a normal healthy couple impregnation follows one connection. So if a couple wanted to limit themselves to three or four or six children, they would be entitled to have relations only three, four or six times in their lives. For it must be remembered that during pregnancy sexual relations would be prohibited, as during pregnancy no further impregnation can take place, and no intercourse must take place which has not for its purpose the conception of a new human being. If the people were believers in big families, and agreed to have twelve children—no anti-Malthusian would expect more than that—they would be entitled to twelve relations during their marital life. Assuming that not every act is followed by pregnancy, but that it takes on the average three or four times to bring about the desired result, we will have it that during the wife's childbearing period the couple may indulge in sex relations from once in three or four years to once or twice a year.

Can a sane person knowing anything about the sexual instinct make any such demands from married people living in the same house and perhaps occupying the same bed? It must be borne in mind that as soon as the wife has reached the menopause all relations must cease, because she can no longer become pregnant, and intercourse without a probable or possible pregnancy is a sin. Also remember that no matter how beautiful, young and passionate the wife may be, if she has some little trouble which makes pregnancy impossible, sex relations must be absolutely abstained from. And of course if the husband or wife is sterile, all relations must be renounced forever, no matter how strong the libido may be in one or both.

It is strange that Nature did not act according to the formula of our sex fanatics; no pregnancy, no intercourse. If she had meant it to be that way, she would have abolished sexual desire in woman immediately after the menopause. Unfortunately this is not the case. For we know that the sexual libido in women after the menopause is often and for several years stronger than before. Why? Nor has Nature abolished the sexual instinct and the passionate desire for sex relations in all those men and women who are for some reason or other sterile, or otherwise so defective that no child can result from the union.

As I stated at the beginning, it is a waste of time to *argue* the matter. Those who believe that sex relations are for racial purposes only, are welcome to their belief, and are welcome to live up to it. (How few of them do, though, honestly and consistently?) We must reiterate our opinion that the sex instinct has other high purposes besides that of perpetuating the race, and sex relations may and should be indulged in as often as they are conducive to man's and woman's physical, mental and spiritual health. No iron-clad rules can be laid down as to the frequency. For some people three times a year may be sufficient, others may require relations three times a month (the best for the average) and still others may not be satisfied with less than three times a week. The human *libido sexualis* cannot be put into an iron mould, and you should pay no attention to religious fanatics who are ignorant of physiology and psychology and who can only blunder and bungle up things.

CHAPTER XXXVIII

VAGINISMUS

Vaginismus—Dyspareunia—Difference Between Vaginismus and Dyspareunia—Adherent Clitoris a Cause of Masturbation and Convulsions.

By the term vaginismus we understand a painful spasm or contraction of the vaginal orifice which makes intercourse very difficult, or impossible.

Certain cases of vaginismus, or rather false vaginismus, may be due to laceration or inflammation of the vaginal orifice, but in genuine cases of vaginismus no local disease can be found, because genuine vaginismus is of nervous origin.

Dyspareunia means painful or difficult intercourse, from whatever cause. It differs from vaginismus in that the cause is generally a local one, that is, it may be inflammation, laceration as after a confinement, small size or atresia of the vagina, etc. When vaginismus is present, it is present in reference to all men, in fact the mere touch of the finger or an instrument may call forth a painful spasm; while dyspareunia may show itself with one man and be absent with another. The origin of the word dyspareunia shows that this may be the case, for *dyspareunos* in Greek means badly mated.

Dyspareunia must not be confused with true vaginismus. In dyspareunia the sexual act can be freely indulged in, only the act is painful or disagreeable. In vaginismus intercourse is *impossible*. In exceptional cases where the husband attempts to use brute force, the wife may faint away, she may get a convulsion or become wildly hysterical. If the husband insists in attempting relations, the wife may run away, or in exceptional cases even attempt suicide.

ADHERENT CLITORIS OR PHIMOSIS

The word phimosis means "muzzling," and it is a term applied to a constriction or narrowing of the foreskin, so that the glands of the clitoris cannot be freely uncovered. This condition may give rise to an accumulation of smegma or secretion which may cause inflammation, itching, and nervous irritation. This in its turn may be the cause of masturbation. It is claimed by some that an adherent clitoris may even be the cause of convulsions resembling epilepsy. In some cases it leads to an irritable bladder, inability to retain the urine, and nocturnal bed-wetting.

In all girls, big or little, that show a tendency to masturbate or simply to handle the genitals, or that complain of itching, the clitoris should be examined and if adhesions are found they should be separated. This can easily be done under a local anesthetic.

CHAPTER XXXIX

STERILITY

Definition of Sterility—Husband Should First be Examined—One-child Sterility—The Fertile Woman—Salpingitis as a Cause of Sterility—Leucorrhea and Sterility—Displacement of Uterus and Sterility—Closure of Neck of Womb and Sterility—Sterility and Constitutional Disease—Treatment of Sterility.

Sterility or barrenness is a condition of inability to have children. In former years the opinion prevailed generally, whenever a couple was childless, that the fault was exclusively the woman's. It wasn't even thought that the man could be to blame. We now know that in at least *fifty per cent.* of cases of sterility, or childless marriages, the fault is not the woman's but the man's. It is therefore very unwise in conditions of sterility to subject the wife to treatment without first examining the husband. Nevertheless, this is still often the case, particularly among the lower classes or among the ignorant. There are cases where the woman goes from one doctor to another for years and is subjected to all kinds of treatment, when a simple examination of the husband would show that the fault lies with him.

Some women have one child and are unable afterwards to give birth to any more. Such a condition is called one-child-sterility. It is generally due to an inflammation of the Fallopian tubes which closes up the openings of the tubes into the womb, so that no more ova can pass *from* the ovaries *through* the tubes *into* the womb. This inflammation may be the result of childbirth, for childbirth alone may set up an inflammation, or it may be due to an infection contracted from the husband.

In order to be fertile, that is, to be able to conceive and give birth to a living child, the woman's external and internal genital organs must be normal, her ovaries must produce healthy ova, and there must be no obstruction on the way, so that the ova and the spermatozoa can meet. The mucous membrane of the womb must also be healthy, so that when the impregnated ovum gets attached to the womb it may develop there without any trouble, and not become diseased or poorly nourished and cast off.

We must always remember that the woman's share in bringing forth children and perpetuating the race is much more important than the man's. When a man has discharged his spermatozoa his work is done—the woman's only commences.

The conditions which cause sterility in women are many, but the most common cause is a salpingitis or an inflammation of the Fallopian tubes, which may be caused by gonorrhea or any other inflammation. A severe leucorrhea may also be the cause of sterility, because the leucorrheal discharge may be fatal to the spermatozoa. Another cause is a severe bending or turning of the uterus either forwards or backwards. The opening of the neck of the womb, the os, may also be closed, or practically so, from ulceration, from strong applications, etc. In some cases sterility may be due to severe constitutional disease, when the person is very much run down and so anemic that menstruation stops. Unfortunately this is not always the case, for women even in the last stages of consumption may, and often do, become pregnant. Syphilis unfortunately does not cause sterility; it only causes miscarriages until controlled by treatment.

The treatment of sterility can be successfully carried out only by a competent physician, particularly by one who is devoting himself specially to this kind of work. But I want once more to impress upon every woman who is sterile, and who wants to have a child, not to have herself treated or even examined until her husband has been subjected to an examination.

CHAPTER XL

THE HYMEN

Difference Between Chastity and Virginity—Worship of Intact Hymen—Sacrificing Hymen Sometimes Essential for Health of the Girl—Certificate from Physician who has Ruptured Hymen.

I have mentioned in a previous chapter that the absence of the hymen was no proof of unchastity, just as the presence of the hymen was no proof of perfect chastity. Chastity and virginity are not synonymous, and a girl may possess physical virginity, that is, an intact hymen, and still be morally unchaste. She may be in the habit of indulging in unnatural sexual practices. But the laity does not know these facts or does not want to know them, and the intact hymen is still worshipped like a fetish. This would be of little consequence, if it did not often result in unnecessary suffering to the female child or girl. Much disease and a good deal of sterility result from the fear of tampering with the hymen.

When a boy gets some trouble with his genital organs, such as phimosis, or balanitis or whatever it may be, he is at once taken to a physician, who institutes the necessary treatment. When a little girl complains of itching around the genitals or of some discharge, the mother will hesitate long before taking her to a doctor. She will be afraid he will do something to the hymen. And so she will temporize, using salves and washes, and the disease will in the meantime be making progress, that is, getting worse. When she does take her to a physician, and he says that in order to treat the case thoroughly the hymen has to be stretched or opened, the mother will withhold her consent, and the disease will be allowed to progress. I know of many such cases. This is wrong. When the health of the girl demands and her future child-bearing power is at stake, no hesitation should be felt in sacrificing the hymen.

Though in the future the fuss which is now made about the hymen, the excessive veneration in which it is held, will appear ridiculous, and though I consider it foolish and rather humiliating to the girl, nevertheless, now, when the average husband does lay so much stress on the presence of an unruptured hymen, a physician who in the course of an operation or treatment has occasion to cut or rupture the hymen, will do well to give the patient a certificate to that effect. In case any question regarding the girl's chastity comes up in the future, she can prove by the doctor's certificate that her loss of virginity was not due to sexual relations. Of course the relations between husband and wife, or between prospective husband and wife, should be such that no "certificate" should be necessary; but reality differs from the ideal, and in some cases that we know the husband's suspicions were allayed by the doctor's oral or written statement.

This is as good a place as any to emphasize, that if the bride has a very strong, tough and resistant hymen, the new husband should not use brute force in rupturing it. First, because the pain may be too excruciating and this may create in the wife an aversion to intercourse which may last for many months or years—in some cases forever. Second, a severe hemorrhage may result, which may require the aid of a physician to stop. Wherever a case of very resistant hymen is encountered, the husband should make several attempts; gradual and gentle dilatation, with the aid of a little vaseline and not forcible rupture should be the aim; the result will usually be satisfactory. In exceptional cases, a physician may have to be called in. The operation of cutting the hymen is a trifling one.

It is also interesting to know that some wives have sex relations for months and years, and the hymen remains unruptured. Pregnancy may also result with an intact hymen.

CHAPTER XLI

IS THE ORGASM NECESSARY FOR IMPREGNATION?

Suppression of Orgasm by Woman to Prevent Impregnation—Bad Results of Suppression by the Woman—Orgasm: Relation of to Impregnation—A Hypothesis—A Fanciful Hypothesis—Why Passionate Women Frequently Fail to Become Mothers—Advice to Passionate Women who Desire to Conceive.

Among the laity the opinion is quite prevalent that in order for a woman to conceive she must experience an orgasm, she must have had a pleasurable voluptuous sensation during the act. If she has no orgasm, impregnation cannot take place. So sure are some women that this is so that when they want to avoid conception they repress any orgastic feeling; as they say, they don't let themselves go. Which, I will say, by the way, is one of the causes of female frigidity. If you don't habitually permit a certain feeling to develop, if you repeatedly repress it at the very beginning, at its first manifestation, it is apt to atrophy altogether, to become permanently suppressed, or the suppression develops into a nervous disorder.

Among the medical profession no perfect unanimity has been reached as to the rôle of the orgasm in impregnation. Some sexologists like Kisch and Vaerting believe it does play an important rôle; others, like Forel, believe it plays none. That the orgasm is not *necessary* for impregnation admits of no discussion. Women who suffer from frigidity in an extreme degree, women who never experienced an orgasm, women who repress their orgasm, women in sleep or under narcosis, women who have been raped, women who loathe their husbands, become pregnant frequently and readily. But does it play any rôle at all? Does it facilitate impregnation? Other things being equal, will intercourse accompanied by an orgasm be more likely to prove fruitful than one in which the orgasm was entirely absent? This question I am forced to answer in the affirmative. Because from the various investigations I have made it can hardly be subject to doubt that the uterus during an orgasm exerts a certain amount of suction; and that impregnation is *more likely* to follow when the spermatozoa are sucked up into the uterus than when left to make their own way by their own power of motion, stands to reason and goes without saying. In the former instance it takes less time for the spermatozoa to reach the ovum, and there is less chance for them to perish on the way—from malnutrition or from coming in contact with secretions of an acid reaction. There is another point. I do not bring it forth as a proved fact or as a fact susceptible to proof. It is a mere hypothesis, but in my opinion it is a correct and plausible hypothesis. I believe that the strong spasmodic contractions that take place during the orgasm have an influence not only in accelerating the bursting of a Graafian follicle and the extrusion of an ovum, but they are instrumental in aiding the Fallopian tube to grasp the ovum and helping it along on the road towards the uterus. It is therefore not at all inconceivable that conception may take place during or within a very short time after an act which is accompanied by a proper orgasm. Many women claim to experience peculiar unmistakable sensations as soon as conception has taken place, and by calculating the day of probable delivery we know that they are right. Taking therefore all the various data into consideration we are fully justified in saying that while an orgasm or a voluptuous sensation during the act is not at all *necessary* to impregnation, it is in many cases a helpful factor.

It is claimed by some that the offspring resulting from an orgastic act is apt to be healthier and better developed than offspring resulting from sexual intercourse in which the parties experience no orgasm. The reason given being that conception in the first instance taking place quickly, the spermatozoa are better nourished and more vigorous. In my opinion this is merely a fanciful hypothesis which needn't be taken seriously.

It will be found rather frequently that women of strong passionate natures, with strong orgastic feelings, and normal in every way, fail to become mothers. A careful investigation of their menstrual discharge will show that *it is not because they failed to conceive,* but because the impregnated ovum is expelled each time; in other words, they have each month a miniature miscarriage. And these miscarriages, or rather abortions, are due to the spasmodic contractions of the uterus and its adnexae which accompany the orgasm. In such cases I have advised the woman to try to remain passive during the act, to repress the orgasm, and the results have in some instances shown the wisdom of my advice. After conception has taken place, after one period has been missed, the woman should abstain from intercourse altogether or at least for two or three months until the fetus is securely attached to, or ensconced in, the uterus.

CHAPTER XLII

FRIGIDITY IN WOMEN

Meaning of Term Frigidity—Types of Frigidity—Large Percentage of Frigid Women—Repression of Sexual Manifestations and Frigidity—Frigidity and Masturbation—Frigidity and Sexual Weakness of Husband—Frigidity and Dislike of Husband—Organic Causes of Frigidity—A Frigid Woman May Become Passionate—Treatment of Frigidity.

The word frigidity means coldness, and when a woman has no desire for sexual relations or experiences no pleasure when she has sexual relations, she is said to be frigid.

Some cases suffer only from lack of desire, others only from lack of pleasure, and still others from both. In some cases the frigidity is congenital, that is, the lack of desire with inability to experience pleasure during the act is inborn. In most cases, however, it is acquired, or is only temporary, and is due to various causes. Frigidity is much more widespread among women than it is among men. Some physicians claim it is present in fifty per cent. of all women. This may be an exaggeration, but if we put the number at twenty-five per cent. we will be quite near the truth.

The causes of frigidity in women are many, but here are the most important ones: First and foremost is the repression of all sexual manifestations which the unmarried woman has to practice, and has had to practice for many centuries. So that a part of the frigidity is hereditary. You cannot entirely eradicate a natural instinct, but that by continually repressing it, by giving it no chance to assert itself, you may weaken it—about this there can be no question.

The second cause is masturbation. Cases that have been addicted to excessive masturbation are very apt to develop not only frigidity, but complete aversion to the sexual act, and inability to experience any pleasure or orgasm. Such cases we come across every day.

A third very important cause is sexual weakness in the husband. When the husband is sexually weak (suffering with premature ejaculations) he either fails to awaken the sexual instinct in the woman, or if it has been awakened it is apt to turn not only into frigidity but into aversion to the act.

The fourth cause is often merely dislike towards the husband. The last two causes, weakness of the husband and dislike towards him, are unfortunately very frequent, and a wife who was frigid with one husband may show herself very passionate on marrying another man.

The fifth cause is fear of pregnancy.

The above are the five principal causes. Other causes may be disease of the uterus, laceration of the cervix, inflammation of the ovaries, vaginismus, disease of the thyroid gland, etc.

It is an unfortunate fact that women who were frigid up to the age of forty or so may become very passionate after that age.

As to the treatment of frigidity, little or nothing can be done for frigidity that is congenital. Most of the other kinds of frigidity, however, can be cured.

CHAPTER XLIII

ADVICE TO FRIGID WOMEN, PARTICULARLY WIVES

Advice to Frigid Women—Attitude of Different Men Towards Frigid Wives—Orgasm a Subjective Feeling—A Justifiable Innocent Deception—The Case of a Demi-Mondaine.

I wish to give you a piece of advice which is of extremely great importance to you. I hesitated somewhat before writing this chapter, but the welfare of so many women depends upon following this advice, and I have seen the lives of so many wives spoiled on account of not having followed it, that I decided to devote a few words to the subject.

As you know, about one-third or one-quarter of all women (in other words, one out of every three or four) are sexually frigid. They either have little or no sexual desire, or if they do have, they experience no voluptuous sensation during the act, and never have an orgasm. If you are unmarried, well and good. But if you are married and happen to belong to the frigid type, then *don't inform your husband of the fact*. It may lead to great and permanent trouble. Some husbands don't care. Some are even glad if their wives are frigid. They can then consult their own wishes in the matter, they can have intercourse whenever they want and *the way they want*. They do not have to accommodate themselves to their wives' ways, they do not have to prolong the act until she gets the orgasm, etc. In short, some husbands consider a frigid wife a blessing, a God-sent treasure. But, as I mentioned several times before, in sexual matters every man is a law unto himself, and some men feel extremely bad and displeased when they find out that their wives have "no feeling." Some become furious, some become disgusted. Some lose all pleasure in intercourse, and some claim to be unable to have intercourse with any woman who is not properly responsive. Some begin to go to other women, while some threaten or demand a divorce (of course, such men cannot really love their wives; they may use their wives' frigidity as an *excuse* to get rid of them).

Now, a man has no way of knowing whether a woman has a feeling during the act or not, whether or no she enjoys it, whether or no she has an orgasm. These are subjective feelings, and the man cannot know them unless you tell him. If you belong to the independent kind, if you scorn simulation and deceit, if, as the price of being perfectly truthful, you are willing if necessary to part with your husband or give him a divorce, well and good. You are a free human being, and nobody has a right to tell you what to do with your body. But if you care for your husband, if you care for your home and perhaps children, and do not want any disruption, then the only thing for you to do is not to apprise your husband of your frigid condition. And it won't hurt you to simulate a feeling which you do not experience, and even to imitate the orgasm. He won't be any the wiser, he will enjoy you more, and nobody will be injured by your little deception, which is after all a species of white lie, and is nobody's business but your own. An innocent deception which hurts nobody, but, on the contrary, benefits all concerned, is perfectly permissible.

It may seem rather strange publicly to give advice to deceive and to simulate. And it is undoubtedly the first time that this advice has been given in print. But as I have only one religion—the greatest happiness of the greatest number—I repeat that I can see nothing wrong in advising something which benefits everybody (concerned) and hurts nobody. More than one household which was threatened with disruption was preserved safe and sound by a little simple advice which I gave to the wife, without the husband's knowledge. He was satisfied, and things after that ran smoothly.

Some women are afraid to simulate a voluptuous or orgastic feeling, because they think the husband can discover whether their feeling is genuine or they are only simulating. (Women, and men too, have funny ideas on sexual subjects). This is not so. A notorious demi-mondaine, who was greatly sought because she was known to be so "passionate," confessed that not once in her life did she enjoy intercourse or experience an orgasm. But her mother, who also suffered with absolute frigidity, taught her to simulate passion, telling her that in that way she could make barrels of money; which she did.

It is deplorable that wives—or husbands—should ever be obliged to have recourse to deception or simulation; perfect frankness should be the ideal to be striven after. But under our present social conditions and with the present moral code, an occasional white lie is the lesser of two evils; it may be the least of a dozen evils.

CHAPTER XLIV

RAPE

Definition of Rape—Age of Consent—Unanimous Opinion of Experts—Exceptional Cases—False Accusation of Rape Due to Perversion—Erotic Dreams Under Anesthesia Causing Accusations Against Doctors and Dentists.

Having intercourse with a woman by force, without her consent, is called rape. When the woman is not in a condition to give consent, as when she is insane, feebleminded, unconscious or drunk, or when she is not of the age at which she can legally give consent, it also constitutes rape, and the punishment is the same. The age of consent differs in different countries and in different States, but as a rule is between sixteen and eighteen years. That is, if a girl under the legal age of consent should give her consent or even if she should urge the man to have intercourse with her the man would be punished just as if he had committed rape.

The punishment for rape is very severe in all civilized countries and ranges from ten years' imprisonment to life imprisonment, while in some States in this Union the punishment is death.

It is not my intention to go into an exhaustive discussion of this painful subject. In this brief chapter I merely wish to bring out two facts.

First, that it is the almost unanimous opinion of all experts that it is practically impossible for a man to commit rape on a normal adult girl or woman if she really offers all the resistance of which she is capable. Of course, if the man knocks the woman down with a blow, rendering her unconscious, that is a different matter. But where no brutality is used by the man, and the woman offers all the resistance she is capable of, rape is practically impossible. It is, however, possible that in some cases the girl may be so paralyzed by fear as to be incapable of offering any resistance. When the man threatens her with death or severe bodily injury, then it is rape even if she offers no resistance.

The second point is that it has been established that of the many accusations of rape brought before the courts *most* are false. Out of a hundred cases only about ten are true. The rest are false. This false accusation of rape is due to a peculiar perversion with which some women suffer. Some of the cases are due to hysteria, to imagination, the women really believing that rape or an attempt at rape was committed on them, while investigation shows the accusation to be entirely false. Many accusations of rape are due to a desire for revenge or merely to motives of blackmail.

Careful doctors and dentists will refuse to give laughing gas or another anesthetic to women except in the presence of others, because, as is well known, an anesthetic often causes in women erotic dreams and sensations and makes them believe that the doctor was committing or about to commit an indecent assault on them, and when they come out of the anesthetic they may be so sure of the reality of their dream that they will bring a complaint against the doctor. Many men have suffered disgrace and imprisonment and have had their lives ruined or even paid the death penalty on account of false accusations against them by either pervert, hysterical, revengeful or blackmailing women.

CHAPTER XLV

THE SINGLE STANDARD OF SEXUAL MORALITY

Chastity—Double Standard of Morality—Attempt to Abolish Double Standard—Late Marriages and Chastity in Men—Harmful Advice Given to Young Women—Chastity in Men Not Always Due to Moral Principles—Chaste Men and Satisfactory Husbands—A Statement by Professor Freud—A Statement by Professor Michels—What a Girl has a Right to Demand of Her Future Husband—Three Cases Showing Disastrous Effects of Wrong Teachings.

When a man marries a girl he expects her to be chaste, that is, a virgin, without any sexual experiences. Of men, the same chastity is not expected as a general thing. As long as a man is healthy, free from venereal disease, his previous sexual experiences do not constitute a barrier to his marriage. This is what is known as the double or duplex standard of sex morality.

During the past few years a number of high-minded and well-meaning men and women have been trying to abolish this double standard and to introduce a single standard of morality. That is, they are demanding that the man going to the marriage bed should be just as chaste, just as virginal as his wife is. Whether or no the efforts of these good men and women will ever be crowned with success we will leave open. Whether or no it is even desirable that their efforts *should* be crowned with success we will also leave open. A complete discussion of these questions belongs to a more advanced book on sexual ethics. Here I will merely say that, taking into consideration the fact that the sexual instinct in boys awakens fully at the age of fifteen or sixteen, and that marriage at the present time, particularly among the professional classes, is an impossibility before the age of twenty-eight, thirty, or thirty-five, it seems to be impossible and undesirable to expect that men should live a perfectly chaste life until they enter matrimony, no matter how late that event may take place.

Those who have made a study of the sex instinct in the male seem to think that chastity in normal, healthy men up to the age of thirty or thereabouts is an impossibility, and where it is accomplished it is accomplished at the expense of the physical, mental, and sexual health of the individual. But be it as it may, and leaving disputed questions out of discussion, the fact remains that the vast majority of men of the present day do indulge in sex relations before marriage. And people that are urging upon our young women to refuse to marry men who have not been perfectly chaste are doing our womanhood a very poor service. As it is now, with all mandom to choose from, there are many, too many, old maids. With only ten per cent. to choose from (because it is admitted that at least 90 per cent. of all men have ante-matrimonial relations), what would our women do? They would practically all have to give up any hopes of being married and becoming mothers. And if these ten per cent., who have remained chaste to their married day, were at least a superior class of men in every instance, there would be some compensation in that. Unfortunately, this is far from being the case, because, as all advanced sexologists will tell you, there is generally something wrong with a man who remains absolutely chaste until the age of thirty, thirty-five or forty. It isn't moral principles in all cases; it is mostly cowardice, or sexual weakness. And sad as it may be to state, these perfectly good, chaste men do not generally make satisfactory husbands, and their wives are not apt to be the happiest ones. I fully agree with Professor Freud in his statement "that sexual abstinence does not help to build up energetic, independent men of action, original thinkers, bold advocates of freedom and reform, but rather goody-goody weaklings." And still more to the purpose is the statement of Professor Michels, who says:

"The desire that one's daughter may marry a man who, like herself, and on an equal footing, will gain in marriage his first experience of the most sacred mysteries of the sexual life, is one which *may lead to profound disillusionments*. Even if to-day the demand for chaste young men is extremely restricted, the supply is yet more so, and the article *is of such an inferior quality* that in actual practice the attempt to satisfy this desire is likely to lead to results which will fail altogether to correspond to the hopes inspired by a contemplation of the abstract idea of purity. Many physically intact individuals of both sexes *are far more contaminated* than those who have had actual sexual experience. Others again, superior in the abstract, and from the physically sexual aspect, are *ethically inferior to the unchaste*, so that the union with these latter would be more likely to prove happy than a union with those who are nominally pure." And further, "Careful fathers of marriageable daughters, who seek this virginity in their sons-in-law, will, if they find it, seldom find it a guarantee for the simultaneous possession of solid moral qualities."

All a girl has a right to demand is that her future husband be in good health, physically and sexually, and that he be free from venereal disease. His previous sexual life, provided he is a man of fine moral character in general, is no concern of hers. Even if the man was unfortunate enough to have contracted gonorrhea, that fact should constitute no bar to marriage, provided he is completely cured of it. The only exception is that of syphilis. The girl has a right to refuse absolutely to enter into union with any man who has been infected with syphilis unless she is willing, and does it with her eyes open, to live her life without any children. In syphilis we can never give an *absolute guarantee* of cure and we have no right to subject a woman to any danger of infection with syphilis, be the danger ever so slight, without her knowledge and consent.

DISASTROUS EFFECTS OF WRONG TEACHINGS

What disastrous effects wrong teaching which inoculates the minds of our women with wrong ideas may have, the following three cases reported briefly in *The Critic and Guide,* will show:

Case One was a girl of twenty-four, of well-to-do parents, a college graduate. She was engaged to a really very nice, sympathetic young man, who undoubtedly would have made her an excellent husband. But during her last two years in college she became imbued with the single standard stupidity, and "chastity for men, votes for women" became her slogan. She asked her fiancé if he had been absolutely chaste before he met her. He did not want to play the hypocrite, and he told her the truth that he had not. But he assured her that he had never been infected and that his general and sexual health was in excellent condition. Being then in an exalted mood, she impulsively broke the engagement, declaring that her husband will have to be as "pure" as she was. She soon regretted her step, because she loved the man; but pride did not let her take the initiative towards a reconciliation, and in the meantime her former fiancé fell in love with and married another girl. After four years had passed, and she was in danger of becoming an old maid, she married a man considerably beneath her socially and intellectually, and in every way inferior to her former fiancé. Her marriage is not a happy one.

Case two is similar to case one, except that the young lady in question—now not so very young—is still living in single blessedness, and the chances of her ever being a wife or even somebody's sweetheart are rapidly vanishing. I might add that her fiancé whom she discarded because of his lack of virginity was a very bright young physician, who is now very successful and very happily married. She I hear is a very unhappy person, in danger of sinking into a permanent state of melancholia. And she had been of a very jolly disposition.

Case three is peculiar in that the fiancé *was* absolutely chaste. She asked him, and he told her that he had never had any relations with anybody and he never had a trace or suspicion of any venereal disease. The young lady was not satisfied. She wanted her fiancé to bring her a certificate from a specialist testifying to that effect. The young man told her that it was foolish, that he would not subject himself to the expense and annoyance of a number of tests when he *knew* that not only did he not have any venereal disease, but that there was no possibility of his getting any. No, that did not satisfy her. She became suspicious. "If you have nothing to fear, why do you object to bringing a certificate?" "I have nothing to fear, but I demand that you respect me and trust me sufficiently to believe that I am telling the truth when I declare a thing with such positiveness. If you do not have that much confidence in me now, our future life does not hold much promise of success." One word led to another, and then he broke the engagement, as any self-respecting man under the circumstances would. He is married, and she is not and probably never will be. Three young lives ruined by perverse teachings.

CHAPTER XLVI

DIFFERENCE BETWEEN MAN'S AND WOMAN'S SEX AND LOVE LIFE

Seemingly Contradictory Statements—Faulty Interpretations of Words Sexual Instinct and Love—Difference in Manifestations of Male and Female Sexual Instincts—Man's Sex Instinct Grosser Than Woman's—Awakening of Sexual Desire in the Boy and in the Girl—Woman's Desire for Caresses—Man's Main Desire for Sexual Relations—Normal Sex Relations as Means of Holding a Man—A Physiological Reason Why Man is Held—Man and Physical Love—Woman and Spiritual Love—Preliminaries of Sexual Intercourse in Men and Women—Physical Attributes—Mental and Spiritual Qualities—Difference Between Love and "Being in Love"—Love as a Stimulus to Man—When the Man Loves—When the Woman Loves—Man's More Engrossing Interests—Lovemaking Irksome to Man—Man's Polygamous Tendencies—Woman Single-affectioned in Her Sex and Love Life—Man and Woman Biologically Different.

In reading books or listening to lectures on sex, you will meet with statements which will seem to you contradictory. One time you will read or hear that the sex instinct is much more powerfully developed in man than it is in woman; next time you will come across the statement that sex plays a much more important rôle in women than it does in men. One time you will hear that men are oversexed, that they are by nature polygamous and promiscuous, while woman is monogamous and as a rule sexually frigid; the next time you will be assured that without love a woman's life is nothing, and you will be confronted with Byron's well-known and oft quoted two lines: Man's love is of man's life a thing apart, 'Tis woman's whole existence.

These contradictions are only apparent and result from two facts: first, that the words sex or sexual instinct and love are used indiscriminately and interchangeably as if they were synonymous terms, which they are not; second, there is failure to bear in mind the essential differences in the natures and manifestations of the sexual instincts in the male and the female. If these differences are made clear, the apparent contradictions will disappear. The outstanding fact to bear in mind is that in man the sex instinct bears a more sensual, a more physical, a coarser and grosser character, if you have no objection to these adjectives, than it does in woman. In women it is finer, more spiritual, more platonic, to use this stereotyped and incorrect term. In men the sex manifestations are more centralized, more local, more concentrated in the sex organs; in women they are more diffused throughout the body. In a boy of fifteen the libido sexualis may be fully developed, he may have powerful erections and a strong desire for normal sexual relations; in a girl of fifteen there may not be a trace of any purely sexual desire; and this *lack* of desire for *physical* sex relations may manifest itself in women up to the age of twenty or twenty-five (something that we never see in normal men); in fact, women of twenty-five and even older, who have not been stimulated and whose curiosity has not been aroused by novels, pictures, and tales of their married companions, may not experience any sexual desire until several months after marriage. But while their desire for actual sexual relations awakens much later than it does in men, their desire for love, for caresses, for hugging, for close friendship, for love letters, awakens much earlier than in men, and occupies a greater part in their life; they think of love more during their waking hours, and they dream of it more than men do.

A man—always bear in mind that when speaking of men and women I always speak of the average; exceptions in either direction will be found in both sexes—a man, I say, will generally tire of paying attentions to a woman if he feels that they will not eventually lead to the biologic goal—sexual relations. A woman can keep up with a man for years without any sexual intercourse, being fully satisfied or more or less satisfied with the sexual substitutes—embraces and kisses.

And here is as good a place as any to refer to the notion so assiduously inculcated in the minds of young women, that a persistent refusal of man's demands is a sure way of keeping a man's affections; that as soon as man has satisfied his desires, he has no further use for the girl. This may be the case with the lowest dregs—morally—of the male sex; it is the opposite of true of the male sex as a whole. And I believe that Marcel Prevost was the first one to point it out (in his *Le Jardin Secret*). Nothing will hold a man's affections so surely as normal sex relations. And the cause of this is not, as might be surmised, merely a moral one, the man considering himself in honor and duty bound to stick to the woman whose body he possessed. No, there is a much stronger and surer reason: the reason is of a physiological character. There is born a strong physical attraction which in the man's subconsciousness plays a stronger rôle than honor and duty. Excesses of course must be avoided, for excesses lead to satiety, and satiety is just as inimical to love as is excitement without any satisfaction.

CHOICE BETWEEN PHYSICAL AND SPIRITUAL LOVE

But to return to our thesis: the difference between man's and woman's sex and love life. If a man had to make his *choice* between physical love, i.e., actual sex relations and spiritual love, i.e., love making, kisses, love letters, etc., he would generally choose the former. If a woman had to *choose*, she would generally choose the latter. The man and the woman would prefer both at the same time: physical and spiritual love. But that is not the question. The question is: if it came to a *choice*; and then the results would be as I have just indicated. The correctness of my statements will be corroborated by anybody having some knowledge of human sexuality. A man can fully enjoy sexual intercourse without any preliminaries; with a woman the preliminaries are of the utmost importance, and when these are lacking she is often incapable of experiencing any pleasure. Nay, the feeling of pleasure is not infrequently replaced by a feeling of dissatisfaction and even disgust. A man cares more for the physical and less for the mental and spiritual attributes of his sexual partner; with the woman just the opposite is the case. I am leaving out of consideration sexual impotence, because this is a real disability, and a man suffering with it only irritates the woman without satisfying her. For this she will not stand. But where the man is sexually potent—he may be aged and homely—his other physical attributes play but a small rôle with woman; his mental and spiritual qualities count with her for a good deal more. While a woman may be able to give a man perfect sexual satisfaction, and she may have an angelic character, if her body is not all that could be desired, the man will be dissatisfied and unhappy.

LOVE IN MAN OCCUPIES SUBORDINATE PLACE

Try as we may, we cannot get away from the fact that in man's life love occupies a subordinate place. I am speaking now of love, and not of "being in love." Being in love, as pointed out in another place, is a distinctly pathological phenomenon, akin to insanity, and when a man is in love it may engross every fiber of him, it may preoccupy every minute of his waking hours, he may neglect all his work and shirk all his duties, in fact he is apt to make a much bigger fool of himself than a woman is under similar circumstances. He is less patient, he has less control over himself, he is less able to suffer, he is less capable of self-sacrifice. But this, as I said, all refers to "being in love," which is an entirely different thing from loving. A man may love ever so deeply, and if his love is reciprocated he will go on with his work in a smooth, unruffled manner. He will do better work for it—love is a wonderful stimulus—but he will be perfectly satisfied if he sees his love for an hour or two every day, or even once or twice a week. And if he has important and interesting work to do, he can part with his love for three months or six months without his heart breaking. Not so with woman. A woman who loves considers every day on which she does not see her lover a day lost. And she is apt to be unhappy and inefficient in her work on such days, and she bears separation with much greater difficulty than does man. I do not think that this is due to the fact that a woman's love is always more intense than a man's; no. But he usually has other interests which occupy his thoughts and his emotions, while most women's thoughts and emotions are centered on the man they love. When a woman loves, she could and would spend all her time with the man she loves. She would never tire of love making (I am not referring here to sex relations), or merely of being in the man's proximity. To woman love is a cloyless thing. Man distinctly does tire. No matter how much he may love a woman, too much lovemaking becomes cloying to him, and he wants to get away. Even mere proximity, if too prolonged, becomes irksome to him, and he begins to fret and fidget, and pull at his chains, even if the chains are but of gossamer. Woman should know these facts and act accordingly.

POLYGAMOUS TENDENCIES IN MAN

We now come to the last point in our discussion: the polygamous or varietist tendencies in the male versus the monogamous tendencies in the female. No matter what our moralists, who try to fit the facts to their theories instead of fitting their theories to the facts, may say, the fact remains that man is a strongly polygamous or varietist animal. That many men live through their lives without having had relations with any women except their wives is cheerfully admitted. I assert this in spite of the incredulous smiles of all the cynics and roués in the world. I have known personally a great number of such men. But that they do it without any struggle, and in some cases a very severe struggle, is emphatically denied. And that hundreds of thousands of men are unequal to the struggle—or do not care to engage in any struggle—and live a sexually promiscuous life— anybody who knows anything about life as it is will testify. And his testimony will be corroborated by the reports of the vice commissions and the statements of disreputable-house keepers. To a great percentage of men a strictly monogamous life is either irksome, painful, disagreeable or an utter impossibility. While the number of women who are not satisfied with one mate is exceedingly small.

A man may love a woman deeply and sincerely and at the same time make love to another woman, or have sexual relations with her or even with prostitutes. It is quite a *common* thing with men. It is quite a rare thing with women, though it may happen. As iterated and reiterated time and again, there are always exceptional cases, but we are speaking of the average and not of the exception. The *rule* is that in her sex and love life woman is much more loyal, much more faithful, much more single-affectioned than is her lord and master— man.

Is she on account of it better than, superior to, man? It is futile to speak of better or worse, of superior or inferior. This is the way they are. This is the way man and woman have been made by nature, by a thousand centuries of heredity, by a thousand centuries of environment. The differences lie in biological roots, and it is futile to fight and rail against nature and biology. The proper thing to do is to recognize the facts and make the best of them. To act the part of the ostrich, deliberately to ignore facts which are not pleasant, may be easy, but is it wise?

CHAPTER XLVII

Maternal Impressions

Wide-spread Belief in Maternal Impressions—No Single Well-authenticated Case of Maternal Impression—Birth of Monstrosities—Ridiculous Examples Given by Physicians—So-called Shock Often a Product of Mother's Imagination—Four Cases of Alleged Maternal Impressions—Mother's Health During Pregnancy May Have Effect Upon Child's General Health.

It is believed by many people that strong impressions made upon the mother during pregnancy may produce marks or defects in the child. This belief dates from earliest antiquity, and is widespread among all races. The belief particularly refers to the emotions of fright or sudden surprise; thus it is believed that if a woman during pregnancy should be frightened by some animal, the child might carry the mark of the animal upon its body, or it might even be born in the shape of the animal. Thousands of such *alleged* cases are given in proof. There is hardly a layman, or, particularly, a laywoman, who does not claim to know of authentic cases of maternal impressions.

It is a thankless task to try to shatter well-established beliefs, and I do not hope to succeed in persuading all my readers that all the stories and examples of maternal impressions are untrue and lack scientific foundation. But I consider it my duty to state my belief, whether you accept it or not. In my opinion there is not a single *well-authenticated* case of maternal impression. There is hardly a case of defect or monstrosity where the cause is supposed to be due to maternal impression, which cannot be explained in some natural way, or simply by accident. Thousands of women are frightened or shocked by disagreeable sights, by crippled men, by animals, and still their children are born perfectly normal. On the other hand, many marked, or defective, or monstrous children are born in which no maternal impressions can be given as the cause. So why can it not happen when the mother was frightened by something during her pregnancy, and the child was born with some mark or defect, that the latter was simply an accident and not the *result* of the impression? Because a thing *follows* another thing it does not mean that it was *caused* by that other thing.

Many of the cases given as examples, and by physicians too, are so ridiculous that no scientific man can give them the slightest credence for one moment. When a physician (Dr. Thomas J. Savage) tells us that he attended a lady who had been frightened by a large green frog at or about the middle of pregnancy, and that she gave birth to a monstrosity, the head of which was that of a large frog in shape, with the eyes and mouth and even the coloring of a frog, then he is either telling an untruth, or he shows himself as ignorant and credulous as any illiterate old woman can be. The doctor should know that at the middle of pregnancy the child is *fully formed* and that there is no possibility of an already formed human being changing its shape into that of an animal. Another example given by the same doctor, and showing the calibre of his mentality, is that of a child which, when an infant, not old enough to walk, "would crawl over the floor and pick up little objects such as pins, tacks, small beads, without the slightest difficulty or fumbling." The reason for this "remarkable" skill the good doctor ascribes to the fact that four months before the birth of this child the mother had an outing in the woods and had derived great enjoyment from gathering hickory nuts which she found scattered among the leaves with which the ground was thickly covered!

Very often the so-called shock or fright which the mother experiences during gestation is simply a product of her imagination. We know of many cases where the mothers never mentioned that anything happened to them, and only after the child was born with some kind of mark or defect they began to hunt for causes and claimed that such and such a thing happened to them while they were pregnant, but on close investigation the alleged event was found to have originated in the mother's brain.

In short, while the subject of maternal impressions is an interesting one and demands further investigation, there is at the present time no scientific justification for the belief in maternal impressions. Particularly must we scout any stories of maternal impressions during the latter part of pregnancy, during the fifth, sixth, seventh, eighth, or ninth month. Because after the child is fully formed no mental or psychic impressions can make birthmarks on it, amputate its limbs, or convert it into any sort of monstrosity.

After the above was written and ready for the printer I came across four cases of alleged maternal impressions in a book by Laura A. Calhoun ("Sex Determination and Its Practical Application"). The first three cases the author relates without any comment, taking them evidently for pure coin. The fourth case the lady investigated, and she is frank to say that what seemed at first as a clear case of maternal impression was nothing of the kind but merely a case of heredity. In order to break the monotony for a little while I will reproduce here the four cases in the lady's own words.

The first was that of "a mother who, during pregnancy, was obliged for a certain continuous time to eat sheep's flesh. She took such a sudden abhorrence and distaste of the meat that she only ate it rather than go meat hungry. After the birth of her baby she recovered from this spasmodic distaste of this particular meat. But the child from its first meat-eating days could not endure the smell or the taste of the sheep's flesh. Whenever the child attempted to eat that meat, the result was always the same—indigestion and want of assimilation, and usually attended with acute indigestion cramps."

In the second case "another pregnant mother's particular 'longing' was for mackerel. Her baby was born with what seemed to be the outlines, in a brownish color, of a mackerel on its side, and which design never faded in after years, and the child's ability to eat and digest mackerel was more than normal."

The third case: "The 'longing' of another pregnant mother was for brains to eat. This was provided for her. But as she was slowly approaching the dish of deliciously prepared food, quivering with delight and with the eagerness of a child to be eating it, a cat sprang to the plate and before she could prevent it ate the brains and licked the plate clean. She wept as a child might have done, and was as unhappy and brokenhearted over this fate of the brains food for which she had waited with such keen anticipation of satisfaction as a little child might have been. Shortly after that the little baby was born, and upon one of its shoulder-blades was a representation of the mess of brains, designed in brownish outlines, and which did not fade as the child grew up."

The fourth case: "There lived in a little house in the midst of a flower garden, that in its turn gave into a wide-spreading orchard, a loving and loyal husband and wife with their firstborn child. The wife was now in the first months of pregnancy with her second child. Their nearest neighbor was a Mexican family, among the members of which was a dashing young man of about twenty-two. He and his sister and mother were frequent visitors to this little household of three. But the young Mexican was the most frequent, and the husband's being home or not did not disconcert him. Men of affairs must need spend morning hours, and sometimes afternoon hours, too, inside of offices, but wealthy and aristocratic young Mexicans ride horses all day, decked out with silver, leather, and velvet trappings, both horse and rider. It was this lady's custom to walk among her flowers and fruit trees. And it became the custom of this young caballero to suddenly appear before her during these promenades. Her startled eyes would no sooner perceive the vision of his blazing, dark eyes fastened upon her, than by one pretext and another she made him understand that he was dismissed, and would herself retire into the house. When she would be about to open a gate, suddenly and unexpectedly the young Mexican would appear on the other side and with gracious suavity open the gate, always his passionate, dark eyes upon her, though his words were reserved and polite. If the husband were present, it was still the same. By every means possible he would prolong his stay.

One summer day this lady was lying on her couch on the veranda, sleeping, her eyes covered over. At that time she was having an eye malady that was epidemic in that part of the country. She heard footsteps approaching, but did not disturb herself, as she supposed it was her husband. After some time she suddenly threw off the covering from her face, and there to her astonished eyes stood the young Mexican, intensely looking down upon her with deep concern. At that moment the husband arrived, and the young man told him of a weed growing in that locality that he said would cure the eye malady. When the leaves of this plant were crushed there oozed a yellowish milk; with about a half-dozen applications of this milk to the sore eyes they were healed.

After that the young caballero would ride up and down, Mexican fashion, in front of the house, drawing rein whenever he could get a glimpse of the lady or a word with her. This never failed to annoy her, and also to strike a sudden, sharp terror into her heart. Always his appearance was most unexpected, and always accompanied by the rapt, passionate, dark gaze. Though he was a most clean-souled young man.

Afterward, when the baby was born, one of the child's eyes was marked by the color and fire of the dashing Spaniard's eyes, while its other eye was a calmish blue-gray eye. This was all the more remarkable as neither of the parents of the child had such eyes. Was it a case of maternal impression?

Upon investigation I found that the grandparents of the baby's mother had just such eyes as the baby. The grandfather's were big, dark, flashing eyes, and the grandmother's the mild, blue-gray eyes. So 'bang!' went the theory of mental impression, and in its place came the physical law of reversion."

I do not wish to be misunderstood as claiming that a mother's condition during pregnancy has no effect on the child, and that she need therefore take no precautions and pay no particular attention to her health and her feelings. This is not so. But what I do want to convey is this: That if a mother's health during pregnancy is bad, if she is a prey to worry and anxiety, if she was subjected to great fright or to a shock, then the child's general health may suffer. It may be stillborn, or the mother may have a miscarriage. But it will not produce those specific marks, deformities and monstrosities which are commonly supposed to be the results of maternal impressions.

If I lay somewhat special stress upon the subject of maternal impressions, it is because I pity the poor mothers and want to spare them as much as possible unnecessary worry and anxiety. Besides I want them to believe in the truth and not in error.

CHAPTER XLVIII

ADVICE TO THE MARRIED AND THOSE ABOUT TO BE

Marriage as an Ideal Institution—Monogamic Marriage—Some Reasons for Husbands' Deviations—Importance of First Few Weeks of Married Life—Necessity for Understanding at Beginning—Preventing and Breaking Habits—The Wife's Individuality—Husbands Who are Childish, Not Vicious—Wife's Interest in Husband's Affairs—The "Slob" Husband—The Well-groomed Husband—Bad Odor from the Mouth—Odors from Other Parts of the Body—Treatment for Bad Odor from Perspiration—A Beneficial Powder—Advice Regarding Flirting—Dainty Underwear—Fine External Clothes and Cheap and Soiled Underwear—Delicate Adjustments of Sex Act Required with Some Men—Wife Who Discusses Her Husband's Foibles—A Professional Secret—A Case of Temporary Impotence—The Wife's Indiscretion—The Disastrous Result—A Big Stomach—The Wife's Attitude Towards the Marital Relation—Behavior Preliminary to and During the Act—Congenital Frigidity—Prudish and Vicious Ideas About the Sex Act—Sexual Intercourse for Procreative Purposes Only—Fear of Pregnancy on the Part of the Wife—The Remedy—Other Causes—Wife who Makes too Frequent Demands—Sacrificing the Future to the Present—Esthetic Considerations.

Whether marriage in its present form is an ideal institution destined to endure forever, whether it is in need of radical reforms before it can be considered ideal, or whether it has fundamental irremediable defects, are questions which we are not going to discuss here. The fact is that at the present time the greatest part of the adult population of the world is married; and the part that isn't would like to be. And the greater part of civilized humanity living in a state of monogamic marriage, it behooves us to make the best of it, to get out of it the greatest amount of happiness that we can, obviate as much unhappiness as possible, and to do everything in our power to make it permanent. Separation or divorce are remedies of last resort, and people have recourse to them when they are at the end of their tether. But the proper thing to do is to avoid the necessity of having to have recourse to them. And I believe that a careful, thoughtful perusal of this chapter will help husband and wife to get along better, to avoid unnecessary friction and to retain the mutual physical and spiritual attraction which we call Love for a longer period than might otherwise be the case.

I have the confidence and listen to the intimate confessions of more men and woman probably than any other physician in America, or perhaps in the world. For reasons easily understood they tell me things which they would not think of telling to their regular physician. I have learned of many of the reasons, which in many families led first to a coolness, then to an estrangement, or to quarrels, to separation and divorce. I know the first steps which in many instances draw the husband to another woman. And I wish to tell you, that while I firmly believe in the polygamous or rather varietist tendencies of the average man, nevertheless I am convinced that one of the great reasons why so many married men patronize prostitutes, or have mistresses or lady friends, is to be found in the wives themselves. Many wives *drive* their husbands to other women, and are alone responsible for their suffering, for the cooling of their husbands' affections, and perhaps even desertion. And in the following pages I will endeavor, as stated before, to point out some of the rocks and shoals on which the matrimonial bark is so often shattered, and to offer the wives some suggestions which will help them to retain their husbands' affections and perhaps even also their fidelity.

While the advice is intended primarily for wives, there will be found here and there a salutary piece of advice for husbands. Some of the advice is applicable to both partners, and as to those suggestions which concern the husband only—it will be a good thing for the wives to call their husbands' attention to them.

The first few weeks or the first few months are the most important in the life of a married couple. The stability of the marriage, the future happiness, often depend upon the things which are done or left undone during the initial weeks of married life. A certain understanding must be reached from the very beginning. If your husband does certain things which displease you and which you know should not be done, it is best to say so at the very start. It is easier to prevent the establishment of a habit than to break a habit after it has been established.

Retain Your Individuality. The first piece of advice I have to give you is: *Retain your individuality.* It is a trite but perfectly true observation that altogether too many men who during courtship were chivalry personified assume a dictatorial tone as soon as the knot has been tied. They think that the wife has actually ceased to exist as a separate human being, that she has been absorbed, and with the loss of her name she has lost all right to have her own opinions, her own tastes, and, of course, her own friends. Friends who are obnoxious to one of the marital partners one must give up sometimes; but do not permit your entire personality to be obscured. Explain to your husband that you are still an independent living human being. I do not say, you should at once start a fight. Nothing is more offensive to me than the militant, pugnacious woman, who wears a chip on the shoulder and is continually ready to insist on her "rights." But with gentleness and firmness much can be accomplished. And you want to remember that many husbands act the way they do, not because they are vicious, but because they are stupid or childish. Sometimes it is mere thoughtlessness. They have been brought up wrongly, and some of them sincerely imagine that by repressing the wife's personality, by blotting it out, they are acting in her interest. "It is for her own good." A serious talk with a husband will sometimes have a wonderful effect. It may sometimes change entirely the current of his thoughts. Of course if the husband is a cad, a conceited fool, or a brute, you can do nothing with him; but fortunately not all husbands belong to those categories.

Interest in Husband's Affairs. Be interested in your husband's affairs. No matter what your husband's occupation may be, you should possess enough intelligence to be able to understand what he is doing. It is almost unbelievable how little some wives know about their husband's profession or work. It is a bad thing when strange women understand your husband's work better than you do, and when he finds in them more intelligent and more sympathetic listeners. He may go to them for sympathy. If your husband is a scientist or a research worker or a professional man it is not necessary that you be familiar with all the details of his work, but with the general character you should be. And if you can be of assistance to him in his work, if it be only looking up references, compiling tables and statistics or merely typewriting, it will be appreciated by him, and will sometimes help to knit the bonds a bit closer.

There is another important reason for being interested in and understanding your husband's business. When the husband dies—and a man is not infrequently snatched away in the prime of youth and vigor—the wife is often left to the mercies of the cold world, without money and without a profession. If she understands the husband's business she can continue it and remain economically independent. This has reference not only to ordinary business, like stores or agencies, but to more or less specialized occupations, such for instance as publishing. We know the cases of two widows of publishers of medical journals. When their husbands died everybody was commiserating with them: what will they make a living from? But they understood the details of their husbands' business, and they kept right on. And now those journals are financially more successful than they were when the husbands were at the helm.

Wife's Behavior Toward Sexual Relations. I am now coming to a delicate subject. But, delicate though it is, it must be dealt with unflinchingly, because it is probably responsible for more male infidelity than all other causes combined. I speak of the relation of the wife to her marital duties, in other words, to sexual relations. Too many women regard the sexual act as a nuisance, as an ordeal, as something disagreeable to get through with as quickly as possible; they regard the husband's demands in this line as an imposition, as unfair or even as brutal; and their behavior preliminary to and during the act is such as to cool the ardor of any refined and sensitive man. The reasons for this behavior on the part of many wives are manifold; this is not the place to consider them in detail. I will allude to them briefly. One great cause is congenital frigidity. The woman is cold, frigid, has no desire for sex relations and experiences no pleasure, no sensation from them. Such women are not to blame; they are to be pitied. But even they can behave so as not to repel their husbands. (See **Chapter XLIII**).

Another great cause is the vicious, prudish bringing up, by which the sex act is regarded as something unclean, indecent, animal-like, brutal. Such Women need a good "talking-to," and if they are only not natural born fools, one good explanation often fixes matters. On a par with this general prudishness is the infamous idea promulgated by a few semi-insane, mentally decrepit men and women, that sexual intercourse is for the purpose of propagation only. That only when a child is wanted is the relation permissible; at all other times it is a sin, an "act of prostitution," an offense in the eyes of God, etc., etc. Of course if the wife has such ideas the husband deserves little sympathy. A man should know what ideas the woman entertains whom he is going to make his wife and the mother of his children. But, unfortunately, this, the most important subject of sex and sexuality, is never touched upon by the engaged couple (it would be so indelicate!), and after they are married they often find themselves at opposite poles. Here also a good heart-to-heart talk will do a world of good. I have had several such cases where a little conversation or even a letter saved the couple from disruption.

In many cases the cause of refusal is fear of pregnancy. In this case the wife is right. But the remedy is simple: give her full instruction in the use of contraceptive measures. Other causes are: excessive masturbation, vaginismus, local malformation, inflammation, etc. But whatever the causes of the wife's "bad behavior" may be, they are all amenable to treatment. Some need medical treatment, some psychic treatment, and some nothing but just a common-sense, heart-to-heart talk.

And I would emphasize: Do not repel your husbands when they ask for sexual favors—at least do not repel them too often. Households in which relations are had rather frequently and in which the wives lend their full and eager participation are happier households than those in which the sexual act is indulged in rarely, and with grumbling and side-remarks on the part of the wife.

But of course you should not go to the other extreme either. You should not make too frequent demands upon your husband. With a man the act means a good deal more than it does with a woman; it entails a great deal more of physical and mental exhaustion, and a wife who is unreasonable in this respect is sowing the seeds of discord and unhappiness. She is sacrificing the future to the present. The husband is apt to become afflicted with satiety or impotence—and the wife may have to lead a life of continence for much longer than she would have had to if she had been moderate. In no department of life is moderation so important as in sex life. Non-use, insufficient use and excessive use are all bad. A mutually joyful, eager and moderately frequent participation in the sexual act will contribute most to a happy and long life.

Dainty Underwear. This may be considered too delicate or too trifling a subject to discuss in an important sex book. But nothing is too delicate or too trifling that concerns human happiness, and you will believe me if I tell you that nice underwear or dainty lingerie plays a very important rôle in marital life. And every married woman should have as fine and as dainty underwear as she can possibly afford. A fine or elaborate nightgown may be more important than an expensive skirt or hat. Unfortunately too many women ignore this fact. Externally they will be well dressed, while their petticoats, drawers and undershirts will be of the commonest quality and of questionable freshness and immaculateness. And if anything in a woman's toilet should be immaculately fresh and clean it is, I emphasize, her underwear. Silk and lace and delicate batiste should be preferred, if they can be afforded, and attention should be paid to the color. As a rule, a delicate pink is the color that most men prefer. The sex act with some men requires the most delicate adjustments, and the condition of the underwear may determine the man's desire and ability or inability to accomplish the act. I therefore repeat: whether you are newly married or have been married a quarter of a century, be sure that your underwear is the very best that your means will allow you, and that it is always sweet, fresh and dainty. It will help you to retain the affection of your husband. I know that some allegedly wise ones will scoff at this statement. They may say that an affection that may be influenced by the kind and condition of underwear is not worth having or retaining. But what do these wise ones know! What do they know of the numerous subtle influences which gradually either strengthen or undermine our affections? Follow this advice and you will be grateful.

Do Not Offend Against Esthetics. Some women think that because they are married to their husbands they owe the latter no esthetic consideration. Things that they would be horrified to let a stranger see they do before their husband's eyes without hesitation. For instance, not to beat about the bush, though the subject is not a pleasant one, they will urinate in their husbands' presence, or they will let him see their soiled menstrual napkins, etc. Some husbands may not mind it; but some men are very sensitive—men on the whole are more esthetic than women—and an indifference towards the wife may have its origin in some vulgar or unesthetic procedure on the wife's part. The sexual act, as mentioned before, is a very delicate mechanism, and it is very easy to disarrange it. The act of micturition before the man is known in many instances to have instantly abolished the man's sexual desire which was present before. And a man told me that because he noticed in a closet a lot of rags soiled with menstrual blood he was unable to enjoy relations with his wife for several months. You may think that these are all small things, but life is made up of little things, and many a married life went smash on account of disregarding the little things.

A High Stomach. Avoid if you possibly can a high stomach, or a big stomach, or what we call in technical language a pendulous abdomen. Nothing is more fatal to woman's beauty—and to man's love—than a big stomach, and particularly a hang-down stomach. It at once takes away her youthfulness and makes her matronly—and matronliness is fatal to romance. It is not so much general stoutness that is objected to—some men, as is well known, prefer plump, stout women. And there are some savage tribes in which the preference is given to obese women with enormous abdomens, but this is not the case with the Caucasian race—not in civilized countries, at any rate, and surely not in the United States. First, reduce your carbohydrates, use massage and hydrotherapy, walk for hours at a time, but reduce your big abdomen—or, still better, don't let it get big. Prevention here, as elsewhere, is much better than cure.

Bad Odor from the Mouth. I know of no other physical ailment which is so dangerous, so fatal to the permanency of the love relation as is a strong, offensive odor from the mouth. As a noxious gas blights a delicate plant, so will a strong bad odor blight the delicate plant of love. Yes, a strong malodorous whiff will cool the most ardent passion. The public would be astounded if it knew how many cases of separation and divorce are due to nothing else but a bad odor from the mouth. Therefore, if you happen to suffer from this unfortunate ailment, lose no time in applying to a competent physician, and do not tire of treating yourself, no matter how irksome and time-consuming the treatment may be, until you are completely cured. It is important to your happiness.

Odors from Other Parts of Body. Odors from other parts of the body should be conspicuous by their absence. Normally no artificial aids are needed. Frequent bathing and general cleanliness are alone sufficient. The natural feminine odor—*odor feminae*—is pleasant, attractive and needs no disguise. But where an unpleasant odor from the genitals, feet or armpits is present the proper treatment should be applied, and in such cases the use of a delicate perfume, sachet or scented talcum powder, is quite permissible. Not only permissible but advisable.

A very good treatment for perspiration and bad odor from the feet is the following: bathe the feet night and morning in a basin of water to which has been added an ounce (two tablespoonfuls) of formaldehyde solution. Dry carefully, and then rub in well the following powder. It is simple, cheap and efficient:

Salicylic acid	one dram
Boric acid	one ounce
Dried alum	two ounces
Talcum	four ounces

A little of the powder should be shaken into the stockings every morning, and the stockings should be changed very frequently, once or twice a day. This powder is also efficient against perspiration and bad odor from the armpits.

I am not giving any treatment for bad odor from the mouth, for this condition may be due to a great variety of causes. The cause may reside in the nose; it may reside in the mouth, decaying teeth, throat, tonsils. It may be due to a bad stomach, to some disease of the lungs, etc. Sometimes it is due to overeating. What would be of value in one condition might be useless in another. The right thing, therefore, is to go to a competent physician, have him find the cause of your trouble and outline the proper treatment.

Leucorrhea. Some men find themselves *entirely unable* to have sexual relations with a woman whom they know is suffering with leucorrhea. The mere knowledge of the fact takes away their *ability* to perform the act. It renders them impotent. It disgusts them, and disgust is fatal to sexual power. Only to-day I saw in my office a woman who anxiously begged for advice and treatment. She had been married five years. She has always had leucorrhea, from her fifteenth year as far as she remembers. Otherwise she did not suffer. For the first three years or so her married life has been a happy one.

Then in an unfortunate moment she told her husband about her profuse leucorrhea, and instantly she noticed a change in him. He could not fully hide the expression on his face. And since then he ceased to have intercourse with her. He made a few attempts, but they turned out unsatisfactory to both, and she noticed that he was forcing himself, doing it against his will. She took some patent medicines and went to one doctor, but without any results. Now, unless she could be cured, she feared her husband would demand a separation or a divorce. If you have leucorrhea treat it. And remember you need not initiate your husband in all your unesthetic ailments.

Loyalty. Loyalty on the part of the wife is almost as important as fidelity. And it is in the highest degree disloyal for a wife to talk to her female or male friends about her husband's peculiarities, foibles or weaknesses. The husband's—as well, of course, as the wife's—peculiarities should be what we call a professional secret. Just as a physician is forbidden to talk to outsiders about his patient's troubles, so should a wife not talk about her husband, nor a husband about his wife. I know of a case in which a newly married husband was temporarily impotent (and it was the wife's fault, too). She spoke about it in the deepest confidence to a close girl friend of hers. The friend told it in deep confidence to another friend. And so it went around until it reached the husband's ears. From that moment he made no further attempt to have relations with his wife; a coolness resulted, which led to a separation, which still persists. The wife begged forgiveness, but he was unable to grant it—he felt so deeply hurt.

Flirting. Do not flirt. Men are apt to misunderstand you, and you are apt to get the reputation of a loose woman without in any way having deserved it. I do not say that you should always wear a forbidding expression, and should scowl at people who dare to smile at you or otherwise pay homage to your feminine charms. But there is a difference between a friendly expression and flirting. However, when your husband begins to neglect you, then a mild flirtation may be justifiable. It will *always* do your husband good to know that there are other males in the world beside him, and that some of these males find interest in the female whom he considers his permanent and exclusive property.

Slovenly Husbands. Don't let your husband become a slob. That is just what I mean. It is no use mincing words. Some husbands have never acquired the habit—or if they have acquired it they quickly lost it—of regarding their wives as ladies. "She is not a lady, she is only my wife," is a well-known joke, but some men take it not as a jest. Some men think that before their wives they can be as slovenly and unclean as they please. Give your husband to understand that cleanliness and freshness is not a "sex-limited" attribute, and just as a husband wants his wife to be clean and dainty and well-groomed, so a wife may enjoy the same qualities in her husband. Some women are very fastidious, and while they may say nothing to their husbands for fear of irritating them, they may think a good deal.

Carrying Life Insurance. Every husband should carry some life insurance—as much as he conveniently can. This should be the husband's most pleasant duty, particularly so when the wife has no profession of her own and there are small children to bring up. The lack of consideration, the thoughtlessness—I would call it dishonesty—on the part of many husbands who claim to love their wives is simply heart-breaking. Who of us does not know of cases of refined wives with children left absolutely penniless and forced into wage slavery or even into menial service by the negligence of their husbands? Such things happened even to wives whose husbands were making from three to ten thousand a year. Thoughtlessness, carelessness, procrastination—and then it was too late. There is not a man who makes as little as twenty dollars a week who cannot carry some insurance. I was once poor, very poor. And the terrifying thought, What would happen to my wife and two children if I should be taken off suddenly? gave me many a troubled and sleepless night. And when I took out a thousand dollars insurance I felt some relief. But I felt it was inadequate. I therefore made a supreme effort and soon took an additional ten thousand dollars. And I assure you that the annual premium of two hundred and eighty-six dollars was a terrible burden on me. There were times when I felt as if I had to give it up. But I deprived myself of many necessities (there was no question of luxuries) and I paid my premiums regularly. But in compensation I had restful nights. It was soothing to know that if I should be taken away in my earliest youth my equally young wife and two little babies would not be left penniless. I verily believe that an adequate life insurance prolongs a person's life, because it removes the worry about the future of the wife and children.

I repeat, every husband should carry some life insurance. And the habit of the bridegroom presenting the bride with a substantial life insurance policy is a very good one. It is not only a financial protection to the wife; it is also more or less a guarantee of the husband's fair health.

Making a Will. Another point. Every husband should make a will. This is a delicate point about which most wives would hesitate to speak to their husbands, but the husband should attend to the matter himself. A will doesn't shorten anybody's life, but is very convenient in case of a sudden taking off. This is, of course, particularly important if there is some property. If the husband dies without a will, there is endless trouble and red tape for the wife. An executor has to be appointed, she has to give bonds, etc., etc. If the husband leaves a will making his wife sole executrix, without a bond, all trouble is avoided. I assume, of course, that the husband has perfect confidence in his wife's wisdom and integrity. If he has not and there are children, it is just as well to designate some outside executor or executors. But whichever may be the case, it is a good and sensible thing always to have a will properly made out and witnessed.

CHAPTER LXIX

A RATIONAL DIVORCE SYSTEM

A Rational Divorce System—Storms and Squalls—Two Sides of the Divorce Question—Outside Help and Marital Tangles—A Husband who was a Paragon of Virtue—The Case of the Sweet Wife—The Proper Untangling of Domestic Tangles.

Of course, I am in favor of a rational divorce system. The difficulties, the obstacles, the expense, with which divorce is now surrounded in most civilized countries is simply disgraceful. Make marriage harder and divorce easier, has always been my motto. When life together becomes unbearable then it is better for both husband and wife to cut the tie and to get divorced. Divorce is preferable to separation, because both spouses may be able to lead a new and happier life. Where there are no children to be taken care of a simple declaration of husband and wife repeated perhaps after a lapse of three or six months should be quite sufficient for the granting of a divorce. Where there are children the state should make sure that they will be properly taken care of before a divorce is granted. Where only one party demands a divorce the case should be carefully studied by a commission which should include in its personnel physicians and psychologists; and adultery should most certainly not be the only cause for divorce.

Yes, I am for a sensible, rational and easy system of divorce. But I would always recommend care and caution. "Go slow" should be the guiding motto of husband and wife in such cases. There are periods in a married couple's life when further living together seems unthinkable; and still a month or two or a year passes and the husband and wife live happily together and cannot believe that there was ever any friction between them. The couples are very few, indeed, who never went through any squalls or storms, whose lives were not darkened by disagreements, quarrels and apparently irreconcilable antagonisms. But after the storm the sun shone brightly again, and the quarrels were followed by harmony and peace. After that love was intensified. Were divorce a simple matter, a mere matter of declaration, many couples who live now in harmony would have been divorced—to their great regret perhaps.

Yes, there are two sides to the divorce question. But I would summarize it as follows: Where there is a real incompatibility of characters, where there is no love and no respect, then the sooner the couple is divorced the better, and not only for them but for the children also, if there are any. An atmosphere of hatred and mutual contempt is not a healthy atmosphere for the growing children. But where there is merely irritability, outbreaks of temper, or disagreements which if analyzed can be seen to be due to temporary and remediable causes, then "Go slow," "Don't hurry," should be your motto. There will always be time to get a divorce. While if a divorce has been obtained, even if you regret it, you will most likely stay divorced. Many divorced couples, I imagine, would remarry, if they were not ashamed. They fear it would make them ridiculous—and it would—in their friends' eyes.

OUTSIDERS IN DOMESTIC TANGLES

If you have a disagreement with your husband, try to straighten out the tangle yourself. Don't call in outside help. You will regret it. A stranger's paws are too coarse and too unsympathetic to meddle with the delicate adjustments which constitute marital life, and after you have gotten over your disagreement and are again living harmoniously you will be ashamed to look that third party in the face, and you will probably bear a grudge against him—or her.

Altogether outsiders are not fit to mix in the internal differences between husband and wife. It is absolutely impossible for a stranger to know just where the trouble is and who the guilty party is. Sometimes there is no guilty party. Both husband and wife may be right; they may both be lovely people and still together they may form an incompatible, explosive mixture. And then again the party that to outsiders may seem the angelic one may in reality be the devilish one. It is a well-known fact that people who to the outside world may seem the personification of honor and good nature may be very devils at home. I have long ago given up not only meddling in, but even judging, domestic disharmonies. For it is almost impossible for an outsider to judge justly. I knew a husband who was considered a paragon of virtue. And when a clash came between him and his wife everybody was inclined to blame the wife. But it came out later that the husband had certain ways about him which made the wife's life a very torture. And vice versa. I know of another case where the wife was considered the sweetest thing in the world. She had nice ways about her, but she disliked her husband and made his life a hell. With genuine chivalry he bore everything, believing that it was a man's duty to bear his cross. She was unfaithful to him, but she was so clever and cunning that neither he nor anybody else suspected it. The fact became painfully patent to him, when on one of the rare occasions that they came together she infected him with a venereal disease, which incapacitated him for a long time. Nobody knew why he insisted upon a separation, and everybody, with the exception of his physician and perhaps one or two others, was blaming him for an unfeeling brute.

I will therefore repeat that as a general thing domestic tangles should be untangled by the tanglers themselves. It is not safe to call in outsiders—relatives or friends; they are apt to make the tangle more tangled, and, what is more, they are quite likely to put the blame on the innocent party, and bestow upon the guilty party the Montyon prize for virtue and gentleness.

CHAPTER L

WHAT IS LOVE?

Is Love Definable?—Raising a Corner of the Veil—Two Opinions of Love—The First Opinion: Sexual Intercourse and Love—The Second Opinion—The Grain of Truth in Each—The Truth Concerning Love—Foundation of Love—Sexual Attraction and Love—The Frigid Woman and Her Husband—Puzzling Cases of Love—The Paradox—Blindness of Love and the Penetrating Vision of Love—Limits of Homeliness—Physical Aversion and Genesis of Love—Mating in the Animal Kingdom—Mating in Low Races—Love in People of High Culture—Difference in Love of Savage and Man of Culture—Distinctions Between Loves—Varieties of Love and Varieties of Men—"Love" Without Sexual Desire—Refraining and Wanting—Cause of Love at First Sight—"Magnetic Forces" and Love at First Sight—The Pathological Side—Differentiation of Phases of Love—Infatuation—Difference Between "Infatuation" and "Being in Love"—Sexual Satisfaction and Infatuation—Sexual Satisfaction and Love—Infatuation Mistaken for Love—Love the Most Mysterious of Human Emotions—Great Love and Supreme Happiness.

I shall not attempt to give a definition, either brief or extensive, of Love. Many have tried and failed, and I shall not attempt the impossible. Nor shall I attempt to discuss Love in all its innumerable details.[9] To do so would alone require a book many times more voluminous than the one you have before you. I shall, however, endeavor to raise a corner of the veil which surrounds this most mysterious, most baffling and most complex of all human emotions, so that you may get a glimpse into its intricate mechanism and perhaps understand what Love is in its essence at least.

Sexual and Platonic Love. There are two widely different, in fact diametrically opposite, opinions as to what constitutes Love. One opinion is that Love is sexual love, sexual attraction, sexual desire. To people holding this opinion love and sexual desire or "lust" are synonymous. And they laugh and sneer at any attempt to idealize

---

[9] To avoid confusion, I will state here that I am discussing love between the opposite sexes, and not maternal love, homosexual love, love for one's country, etc.

love, to present it as something finer and subtler, let alone nobler, than mere sex attraction. The writer has heard one cynical woman— and more than one man—say: Love? There is no such a thing. Sexual intercourse is love, and that's all there is to it.

The other opinion is that Love, true love, ideal love, or, as it is sometimes called, sentimental love, or platonic love, has nothing to do with sexual desire, with sexual attraction. Indeed, people holding this opinion consider love and sexual attraction—or lust as they like to call the latter—as antithetical conceptions, as mutually antagonistic and exclusive.

Both opinions, as is often the case with extreme and one-sided opinions, are wrong. Both opinions have a reason for their existence, because there is a grain of truth in both of them. But a grain of truth is not the whole truth, and if an opinion contains ninety-nine parts of untruth to one part of truth, then the effect of the opinion is practically the same as if it were all false.

Here is the truth, or at least what I think is the truth, as it appears to me after many years of thinking and many years of observing.

Foundation of Love. The *foundation*, the *basis* of all love is sexual attraction. Without sexual attraction, in greater or lesser degree, there can be no love. Where the former is entirely lacking the latter can have no existence. This you may take as an axiom. Some may call it love, but on analyzing it you will find that it is no such thing. It may be friendship, it may be gratitude, it may be respect, it may be pity, it may be habit, it may even be a *desire* or a *readiness* to love or to be loved, but it is not love. Experience has proved it in thousands and thousands of sad cases. And the girl who marries a man who is physically repulsive to her, who possesses *no* physical sexual attraction for her, though she may experience for him all of the feelings mentioned above, namely, friendship, gratitude, respect and pity, is preparing for herself a joyless couch to sleep on. Unless, indeed, she happens to belong to the class of women whom we call frigid, that is, if she is herself devoid of any sexual desire and feels no need of any sexual relations. Such a woman may be fairly or even quite happy with a husband who repels her physically, but whom she likes or respects. And what I said about the wife applies with still greater force to the husband. A man who marries a woman who is physically antipathetic to him is a criminal fool.

I repeat, sexual, physical attraction is the *basis*, the foundation of love. It is true we see certain cases of love which puzzle us. We cannot understand what "he" has seen in "her" or what "she" has seen in "him." But let us remember this paradox, which paradoxical though it be, is true nevertheless: Love is blind, but Love also sees acutely and penetratingly; it sees things which we who are indifferent cannot see. The blindness of Love helps her not to see certain defects which are clearly seen to everybody else; but, on the other hand, her penetrating vision helps her to see good qualities which are invisible to others. And a homely person may possess certain compensating *physical* qualities—such as passionate ardor or strong sexual power—which, render him or her irresistible to a member of the opposite sex.

But homeliness, ugliness or deformity have their limits, and I challenge anybody to bring forth an authenticated case in which a man fell in love with a woman—or vice versa—who had an enormous tumor on one side of the face, which made her look like a monstrosity, or whose nose was sunk in as a result of lupus or syphilis, or whose cheek was eaten away by cancer. Love under such circumstances is an absolute impossibility, because there is physical aversion here, and physical aversion is fatal to the *genesis* of love. A man who loved a woman may continue to love her after she has become disfigured by disease, but he cannot fall in love with such a woman.

I will repeat, then, and I trust you will agree with me on this point: sexual attraction is the foundation of all love between the opposite sexes. Where sexual attraction is lacking you can give the feeling any other name you choose: it will not be love.

Other Requisites. But a foundation is not a whole structure. To insure the stability of a high intricate building we must give it a good solid foundation; but the foundation does not make the building. That still remains to be built. So sexual attraction is the foundation of all love, but it does *not* constitute love. Many more factors, many more wonderful stones are needed before the wonderful structure called love is brought into existence. This wonderful structure sometimes goes up in the twinkling of an eye, as if by the touch of a magic wand—who has not seen or heard of instances of "love at first sight!"—but the rapidity of the growth of the structure called Love does not militate against our assertion that many stones, much variegated material, and a strong cement are needed for its completion. Fairies sometimes work very quickly.

A little thought will show clearly that Love is not merely sexual love, not merely a desire to gratify the sexual instinct. If love were merely sexual desire, then one member of the opposite sex, or at least one attractive member, would be as good as any other. And indeed in animals and in the lower races, where love as we understand it does not exist, this is the case. To a male dog any female dog is as good as another, and vice versa. Cats are not particular in the choice of their mates, nor are cows, horses, etc. And the same is true of the primitive savage races, and even among the lower uneducated classes of so-called civilized races. To the Hottentot, to the Australian bushman or to the Russian peasant one woman is as good as another. If the male of a low race has some preference, it will be in favor of the woman who happens to have a little property.

In fact I make the assertion that real love, true love, is a new feeling, a comparatively modern feeling, absent in the lower races and reaching its highest development only in people of high civilization, culture and education.

The platitudinous objection might be raised that "human nature is human nature," that all our feelings are born with us, and as such are inherited, that they have been with us for millions of years and that we cannot possibly *originate* any entirely new feeling. True from a certain viewpoint. We cannot originate intellect either. The germ of intellect with all its potential possibilities was present in our most primitive tree-climbing ancestors. But as much difference as there is between the intellect of an Australian bushman and the intellect of a Spinoza, a Shakespeare, a Darwin, a Victor Hugo, a Goethe or a Gauss, so much difference is there between the love of a primitive savage and the love of the highly cultured modern man. The love or so-called love of the primitive or ignorant man (and woman) is a simple matter and is practically equivalent to a desire for sexual gratification. The love of the truly cultured and highly civilized man and woman, while still *based* on sexual attraction, is so complex and so dominating a feeling that it completely defies all analysis, all attempts at dissection, as it defies all attempts at synthesis, at artificial building up.

As previously stated, some writers attempt to make a clear distinction between sensual and sentimental love; many reams of paper have been used up in an endeavor to differentiate between one and the other; the first is called animal love or lust; the second pure love or ideal love; the first variety of love is said to be selfish, egotistic, the other—self-sacrificing, altruistic. These distinctions read very nicely, but they mean very little. There is no distinct line of demarkation between the two varieties of love, and one merges imperceptibly into the other. Most, if not all, of our apparently altruistic actions and feelings have an egotistic substratum; and the quality of the love depends upon the lover. In other words, there are not two separate, distinct varieties of love, but there are separate, distinct varieties of men. A fine and noble man will love finely and nobly; a coarse and brutal man will love coarsely and brutally. A man who is fine and noble may not love at all, but he cannot love coarsely and selfishly; and a coarse and brutal man can never love nobly and unselfishly. Which once more means: the difference is not inherent in the love, but in the lover.

But to say that a man may deeply love a woman and not have any sexual desire for her is nonsense. A man who loves a woman and does not want to possess her (to use the ugly ancient verb) does not love her—or he is completely impotent. Whatever the feeling may be for her—it is not love. He may abstain from having sex relations with her if the circumstances are such that sex relations may lead to her unhappiness and suffering, but to refrain from doing a thing, when reason and judgment lead us to refrain, does not mean not to want the thing.

Love at First Sight. Nothing is more firmly established than the fact that a person may fall passionately and incurably in love with a person of the opposite sex at the very first sight, in the twinkling of an eye, in the literal sense of the word. One glance may be sufficient.

And such a love may exist to the end of life, and may, if reciprocated, lead to supreme happiness, or if unreciprocated to the deepest unhappiness.

What it is that causes love at first sight is unknown. Some have suggested that the beloved object sets in motion or fermentation certain internal secretions (hormones) in the lover which cannot become "satisfied" or "neutralized" except by that person; and the possession of the beloved object becomes a physical necessity. This explanation really means nothing. It is a hypothesis unsusceptible of proof. But whatever the cause of love at first sight, it is so mysterious a phenomenon that it gives the mystics and metaphysicians some justification for their talk about "electric currents" and "magnetic forces." These phrases also mean nothing, but are an attempt at explaining the suddenness and irresistibleness of the attack. So powerful is the attraction of love at first sight that people have been known to cross continents and oceans merely to get a glimpse of the beloved object; and people have been known to sacrifice *everything*—their career, their material possessions, their social standing, their honor, and even their wife and children, in order to gain their object. And a mother may give up her children whom she loves dearer than life, may risk ostracism and disgrace, only in order to be with the object of her love. This shows that love, then, becomes pathological, because any feeling which so completely masters an individual that he is willing to sacrifice everything he has in the world is pathological.

Infatuation and Being in Love. While, as said, the feeling of love does not readily lend itself to dissection, to analysis, still we can differentiate some phases of it. We can differentiate between "being in love," "infatuation," and "love." Being in love is, as just indicated, a pathological, morbid phenomenon. The person who is in love is not in a normal condition. He can see nothing, he cannot be argued with, as far as his love is concerned. She is the acme of perfection, physical, mental, and spiritual; nobody can be compared with her. And, of course, the man is anxiously eager to marry the object of his love—unless insuperable obstacles are in the way; for instance, if the man happens to be married.

Infatuation may be as strong as any "being in love" feeling. But with this difference. In infatuation the man may know that the object of infatuation is an unworthy one, he may despise her, he may hate her, he may pray for her death, he may do his utmost to overcome the infatuation. In short, infatuation is a feeling, chiefly physical, which the man can analyze, the unworthiness and absurdity of which he may acknowledge, but which he is unable to resist or overcome. He feels himself bewitched; he feels himself caught in a net, he is anxious to tear asunder the meshes of the net, but is not strong enough to do it.

And this is a pretty good way to differentiate between being in love and being infatuated. If in love the man does not want to be free from his chains; he does not want to cease to love or to be in love. When infatuated the man often uses his utmost will-power to break his shackles. Sexual satisfaction is often sufficient to shatter an infatuation; it is not sufficient to destroy love—it often strengthens and eternalizes it.

Neither being in love nor infatuation can last "forever"; they are acute maladies of high tension and relatively short duration. Infatuation may change into indifference or disgust; "being in love" may change into indifference, hatred, or into real love—a steady, durable love.

This will answer the often asked question: How do marriages turn out which are the result of a sudden, violent passion, or of love at first sight? No ironclad rules suitable for all cases can be given. Some turn out very unhappily, the couple gradually finding out that they are altogether unsuited to each other, that their temperaments are incompatible, that their views, ideas, likes and dislikes are different. In some cases what was supposed to be a great love is soon seen to have been merely an infatuation. And satiety and disgust follow. But in other cases, as mentioned, the sudden consuming passion turns into a warm, life-long love and the people live happily ever after.

Dr. Nyström relates the case of a prominent physician of France, of high social and scientific standing, who beheld a young girl accidentally in the street. He did not have the slightest idea who she was. He was irresistibly attracted to her. He followed her, boarded the same omnibus and went to the house which she entered, rang the bell, introduced himself, begging pardon for his intrusion, but was dismissed. He returned and explained to her his ardent passion and asked permission to visit her parents, well-to-do people in the country, and the climax was a mutual love and a happy marriage.

Many of us know of similar cases. But as a rule the slow developing love is more reliable than the suddenly bursting out flame.

Love is the most complex, the most mysterious, the most unanalyzable of human emotions. It is based upon the difference in sex—upon the attraction of one sex for another. It is fostered by physical beauty, by daintiness, by a normal sexuality, by a fine character, by high aspirations, by culture and education, by common interests, by kindness and consideration, by pity, by habit and by a thousand other subtle feelings, qualities and actions, which are difficult of classification or enumeration.

A great love, greatly reciprocated, is in itself capable of rendering a human being supremely happy. *Nothing else is.* Other things, such as wealth, power, fame, success, great discoveries, may give supreme satisfaction, great contentment, but supreme, buoyant happiness is the gift of a great love only. Such loves are rare, and the mortals that achieve it are the envy of the gods. But a great love, unreciprocated, especially when admixed to it is the feeling of jealousy, is the most frightful of tortures; it will crush a man like nothing else will, and the victims of this emotional catastrophe are pitied by the inmates of the lowest inferno.

CHAPTER LI

Jealousy and How to Combat It

Jealousy the Most Painful of Human Emotions—Impairment of Health—Mental Havoc—Jealousy as a Primitive Emotion—Jealousy in the Advanced Thinker and in the Savage—Jealousy in the Child—Feelings and Environmental Factors—Essential Factors—Vanity—Anger—Pain—Envy—The Impotent Husband's Jealousy—Anti-social Qualities—The Jealous and the Unfaithful Husband—Means of Eradicating the Evil—Iwan Bloch on the Question—Prof. Robert Michels' Statement—Remark of Prof. Von Ehrenfels—Havelock Ellis on Variation in Sexual Relationships—Advanced Ideas—Woman as Man's Chattel—The Change and the Changer—Teaching the Children—Casting Epithets at Jealousy—Free Unions and Jealousy—Feelings, Actions and Public Opinion—The Adulterous Wife of the Present Day—Jealousy Defeating Its Own Object—Jealousy of Inanimate Objects.

He or she who has been so unfortunate as to experience the pangs—or fangs—of jealousy will readily admit that it is one of the most painful, if indeed *not* the most painful, of all human emotions. The suffering that it metes out to its victims is indescribable. No other single human emotion so affects the body, so upsets the mind, so deranges every function, as does jealousy. The torture that it causes makes the sufferer a truly pitiable object: the complete loss of sleep and complete loss of appetite may result in a serious impairment of the sufferer's health, while the rage it often gives rise to may lead to actual insanity, or at least to great mental disturbance. With good reason has popular fancy pictured this cursed emotion as a green-eyed monster.

Jealousy is a primitive emotion. It is present not only in the primitive races, but even in animals. And being a primitive emotion, we can hardly hope to succeed in eradicating it entirely. Not in the immediate future, at any rate. But we can modify it.

The statement frequently heard that "human nature is human nature" is only a platitudinous half-truth. The fundamental part of human nature—the desire for happiness and the avoidance of suffering—cannot be changed, nor would we want to change it if we could. It would mean the disappearance of the human race. But that many of our primitive emotions can be greatly modified by culture, by new standards, by new ideals of morality, about this there can be no question.

Just as love in modern man is an entirely different feeling from what it was in primitive man, so jealousy in the advanced thinker is a different feeling from what it was in the savage; and by education and true culture it can be modified still further. We hope that in time to come—I will not venture to say how soon that time will be here— this injurious, degrading, anti-social feeling may be entirely or almost entirely eradicated from the human breast.

The primitive desire—and this primitive desire of the race is still fully exhibited by children—is to take possession of everything nice or useful that somebody else has and which we have not. But our education and our cultural standards, including fear of punishment, have so repressed this desire, have put it so deeply in the background, that normal human beings hardly feel it at all.

It is only improperly brought up people, mental defectives and those unable to adjust themselves to their environment who still have this primitive feeling of taking or stealing. And so with many other feelings and emotions; and so with jealousy.

If we, at the very first notice of a manifestation of jealousy by a child, should frown upon it, if we should explain to the child or adolescent that jealousy is a mean, degrading feeling, that it is a feeling to be ashamed of, a feeling to hide and not to show off or even be proud of—as some are now—then jealousy would manifest itself in a much smaller number of individuals, and those unfortunate enough to be attacked by it would try to repress it, to hide it, to overcome it, so that it would eventually become paler and less acute and its consequences would be less significant, less disastrous for both the victim and for the persons concerned. Feelings, let us bear in mind, are not spontaneous things uninfluenced by any environmental factors. Feelings are like plants; under one environment you may foster their growth and make them develop luxuriantly; under another environment you may dwarf their growth and strangle them.

In order to enable us to inhibit the growth of the demon of jealousy, we must learn what its essence is and what factors are favorable to its development.

CAUSES OF JEALOUSY

The essential factor in jealousy is *fear*. Fear of losing the beloved object, fear of losing the person who provides you with sexual satisfaction, or the mere economic fear of losing a material provider. The latter kind of fear is, of course, more often manifested—even though unconsciously—in women. Women who have no love for their husbands are nevertheless often fiercely jealous, because consciously or unconsciously they are afraid that their husbands may desert them for other women, and that they may thus find themselves in a precarious economic condition.

Another factor in jealousy is wounded *vanity*. We do not like to feel that somebody is considered superior to us. This feeling of wounded vanity is present in other varieties of envy or rivalry. A person who loses in a race or gets a lower mark in his examination than his rival may be filled with a feeling of envy and hatred almost equal in intensity to, though never as painful as, sexual jealousy.

Another factor in jealousy is *anger* over loss of what we consider our property. In our present social order the man considers his wife his absolute property, and so does the wife consider her husband. And there is anger that a stranger should dare to rob us or make use of our property, just as there would be anger if a thief came and robbed us of a valuable material possession. This anger or rage part of jealousy is not a sign of love. It is very far from being so. Because it manifests itself also in men and women who have not a particle of love for their spouses; it manifests itself in spouses who have nothing but hatred and loathing for their partners.

Another important factor is *pain*, pain that the person we love has ceased to love us. When we love a person and our love is not reciprocated, we feel pain which may rise to the degree of agony, even when there is no rival in the field. But when a person who loved us has ceased to love us—or we imagine so—and has transferred the love to another person that pain is so much the greater.

I will digress here for a moment to state that the fear that a person has ceased to love us because he loves somebody else is often groundless. It is based upon the erroneous and vicious idea that a man cannot possibly love two women at the same time, or that a woman cannot love two men at the same time. Psychologists, particularly those who have made a special study of sexual psychology, know that this idea is false. They know that love may be directed at the same time towards two or three individuals. They know that a second love not only does not necessarily destroy or diminish a first love, but may deepen and strengthen the latter.

Another element is pure *envy*. Just mean envy that somebody should have what we haven't, or what we have but are in danger of losing. Just as we envy others an automobile, a fine house, a high social position, etc., when we have not got them or have been deprived of them.

A point that I would like to mention is, that if husbands who have become impotent—having lost either the desire or the power, but particularly the latter—become jealous, their jealousy knows no bounds. No strongly potent man ever reaches the same intensity in jealousy as is reached by a sexually weak or impotent man. The knowledge that another man has displaced him and that he himself could not replace that other man *even if he were permitted to* fills him with impotent rage; and, as is well known, impotent rage is always more intense than rage that is potent. Women are free from this kind of rage, because women are never impotent in this sense. (They may be frigid, but they are never devoid of the *potentia coeundi*, except in extremely rare cases of *atresia vaginae* or the absence of the external genitals.)

There are a number of other components which go to make up this "queen of torments" or "king of torturers" jealousy, but those I have enumerated are the essential ones.

What are they? Fear, vanity, anger, envy and pain. None of them admirable qualities, none of them, with the exception of the first and the last, even deserving our compassion. All of them anti-social and anti-individual qualities. Should not everything be done to eradicate such a rank weed, which draws its sustenance from roots each one of which is dipped in poison?

We are told that in our primitive state jealousy was a social instinct; that by killing and keeping away rivals it helped to found and cement the family and to keep it pure. I do not care to enter here into a discussion of this point. But whatever useful rôle jealousy may have played in the remote ages (I doubt that it has), it is now an utterly useless, utterly vicious, utterly anti-social and anti-individual emotion. It is opposed to social life and it destroys individual happiness. And everything possible should be done to smother it, to strangle it, to eliminate it entirely from human life.

Yes, I find no compensation whatever for jealousy; I find no place for it in our modern life and I am in complete agreement with Forel, who calls jealousy "a heritage of animals and barbarians." "That is what I would say," he says, "to all those who, in the name of offended honor, would grant it rights and even place it on a pedestal. It is ten times better for a woman to marry an unfaithful than a jealous husband.... Jealousy transforms marriage into a hell.... Even in its more moderate and normal form, jealousy is a torment, for distrust and suspicion poison love. We often hear of justified jealousy. I maintain that *jealousy is never justifiable*; it is always a stupid, atavistic inheritance, or else a pathological symptom."

But can anything be done to eradicate this agonizing, tormenting emotion? I believe it can, and the ways and means to the eradication of this evil will be found on analyzing its components. We may not be able to destroy all the components; if we destroy the greater part of them much will have been accomplished.

The underlying factors of jealousy are: the primitive instinct, also present in many animals, our ethical and religious ideas and our economic system. The primitive instinct we can repress and modify; we can hardly hope to eradicate it entirely. But our ideas and economic system we can change. It is easier to change ideas than it is a system, and it is with our ideas we should commence.

The first idea we must endeavor to destroy is that it is impossible for a human being to love more than one other human being at the same time. We must show that the love of the modern educated and esthetic man and woman is an exceedingly complex feeling, and that a man may deeply and sincerely love one woman for certain qualities and just as deeply and sincerely love another woman for certain other qualities. Of course, love cannot be measured by the yard or bushel, nor can it be weighed on the most delicate chemical balance. And it may be impossible to determine whether he loves both women exactly alike or he loves one woman more than the other. But that one love does not exclude another, that it may even intensify the other love, that is certain, and is the opinion of every advanced sexologist.

Max Nordau, a man of high and austere ideals, a man whom nobody will accuse of a tendency to licentiousness, says in his Conventional Lies: "It may sound very shocking, yet I must say it: we can even love *several* individuals at the same time, with nearly equal tenderness, and we do not necessarily lie when we assure each one of our passion. No matter how deeply we may be in love with a certain individual, we *do not cease* to be susceptible to the influence of the entire sex."

And Iwan Bloch, than whom no greater investigator in the field of sexology ever lived, asks the question: "Is it possible for any one to be *simultaneously* in love with several individuals?" And he immediately says: "I answer this question with an unconditional 'yes.'" And he says further: "It is precisely the extraordinary manifold spiritual differentiation of modern civilized humanity that gives rise to the possibility of such a simultaneous love for two individuals. Our spiritual nature exhibits the most varied coloring. It is difficult always to find the corresponding complements in one single individual."

Prof. Robert Michels says: "It is Nature's will that the normal male should feel a continuous and powerful sexual attraction towards a considerable number of women.... In the male the stimuli capable of arousing sexual excitement (this term is not to be understood here in the grossly physical sense) are so extraordinarily manifold, so widely differentiated that it is quite impossible for one single woman to possess them all."

Prof. von Ehrenfels wittily remarks that if it were a moral precept that a man should never have intercourse *more them once in his life* with any particular woman, this would correspond far better with the nature of the normal male and would cost him far less will-power than is needed by him in order to live up to the conventional demands of monogamy.

And Havelock Ellis cautiously says: "A certain degree of variation is involved in the sexual relationships, as in all other relationships, and unless we are to continue to perpetuate *many evils and injustices*, that fact has to be faced and recognized."

I have devoted considerable space to this topic, and I have, contrary to my custom, quoted "authorities," because I consider this point of the utmost importance; it is the first step in combating the demon of jealousy. If our wives, fiancées and sweethearts could be convinced of the truth that a man's interest in or even affection towards another member of the female sex does not mean the death of love, or even diminished love, half of the battle would be won. Half of the misery, half of the quarrels, half of the self-torture, half of the disrupted homes, in short, half of the tyrannical reign of the demon of jealousy, would be gone.

We must teach our women and men this truth, teach it from puberty on. We must show them that not every woman can necessarily fill out a man's entire life, that not every woman can necessarily occupy every nook and corner of a man's mind and heart, and that there is nothing humiliating to the woman in such an idea (and *vice versa*). She should be taught to find nothing shameful, painful or degrading in such a thought. I know that these ideas are somewhat in advance of the times, but if nobody ever brought forward any advanced ideas because they were advanced there would never be any advance.

Then we must teach our men that when they marry a woman she does not become their chattel, their piece of property, which nobody may touch, nobody may look at or smile at. A woman may be a very good, faithful wife and still enjoy the companionship of other men, the pressure of another man's hand or—*horribile dictu*—even an occasional kiss.

Then we must teach our men *and* women that there is essentially nothing shameful or humiliating in being displaced by a rival. The change may be a disgrace for the changer and not for the changed one. It does not at all mean that the change has been made because the rival is superior; it is a well-known fact that the rival often *is* inferior. The change is often made, not because the changer has gone upward, but because he has gone downward, has deteriorated. And the changer often knows it himself.

Inculcating those ideas would do away with the feeling of wounded vanity which is such an important component in the feeling of jealousy.

Further, we must teach our children from the earliest age that jealousy is "not nice," that it is a mean feeling, that it is a sign of weakness, that it is degrading to the person who entertains it, particularly to the person who exhibits it. Ideas inculcated from childhood have a powerful influence, and the various ideas exposed above *would* have an undoubted influence in minimizing the mephitic, destructive effects of the feeling of jealousy. People properly brought up will always succeed in controlling or suppressing certain non-vital instincts or emotions on which society puts its stamp of disapproval, which it considers "not nice" or disgraceful.

I am, therefore, an optimist in relation to the eventual uprooting of the greater number of components of the anti-social feeling of jealousy. And when woman reaches economic independence, then another component of the instinct of jealousy—the terror at losing a provider and being left in poverty—will disappear.

Jealousy Not Toward Rivals. Jealousy need not express itself toward a sexual rival only. A person may be jealous of people who can never be sexual rivals; the jealousy need not even be of people; it may be of inanimate objects, of a person's work, profession or hobby. Thus a wife may be intensely jealous of her husband's mother, towards whom he is very affectionate or simply kind and considerate. She may be jealous of her own children if she notices or imagines that the father loves them intensely, or if he spends a good deal of time with them. She may be jealous of his male friends, and many a husband had to give up, not only his female acquaintances, but his life-long male friends—in order to preserve peace in the family. A wife may be fiercely jealous of her husband's success and reputation, and cases are not unknown where the wife put every possible obstacle in her husband's way, in order to make him fail in his work, to make him turn out mediocre work, all from fear that his success would gain him admirers, which might perhaps take him away from her. Wives have been known to do everything in their power to *exhaust* and weaken their husbands, to make them physically unattractive, only to keep them. And so powerful is this primitive, childish, savage feeling, this desire for exclusive monopoly, that there is *nothing* a jealous wife, sweetheart or mistress may not do in order to retain the man, in order to regain him, or, having lost him irretrievably, in order to revenge herself. And what is said about the woman is applicable with equal force to man. It is a huge mistake to assume that jealousy is woman's prerogative, her particular characteristic, or even that it is stronger in her than in man. A man can be as savagely jealous as any woman and suffer the same tortures of hell.

Jealousy Defeats Its Object. One of the worst features about jealousy is that it defeats its own object. We have been told, as stated before, that jealousy was once upon a time a racial instinct, that by frightening away rivals it helped to found the family and to keep it chaste and pure. Quite the contrary is true now. More than one man has, by accusing his innocent wife of infidelity and by torturing her with baseless suspicions, driven her into the arms of a lover. We are all more or less susceptible to suggestion, and by continually suspecting a wife of a love affair or illicit relation a man may implant the seed of suggestion so strongly that it may grow luxuriantly and the wife may be unable to resist the suggested temptation. And very often the very lover is suggested by the husband. "Yes, don't attempt to deny it. It is useless. I know you have relations with X. I know you are his mistress." He kept on repeating it so often to his absolutely blameless, innocent young wife and he made her so wretched by his rudeness and brutality that one day she did go over to X's rooms and did become his mistress. And after that she could stand her husband's outbursts with equanimity. "If I have the name I might as well have the game," is a good bit of psychologic wisdom. And a husband should be very careful about even suspecting a wife unjustly, and thus make the first step towards rendering his baseless suspicions a reality, his unjust accusations justified. And, of course, what is true of the husband is also true of the wife. Many a wife has driven her indolent husband into the hands of prostitutes or mistresses by her incessant nagging, false accusations and vicious epithets applied to all his female friends and acquaintances.

Yes, from whatever angle you consider it, jealousy is a mean, nasty, miserable feeling. Because it is a more or less universal feeling, because "we cannot help it," does not render it less mean, less nasty, less miserable.

I do not for a moment imagine that characterizing jealousy the way it deserves to be characterized, calling it a shameful, savage, primitive feeling, etc., is at once going to banish it from the breasts of men and women in which it has found an abiding place; throwing epithets at it will not cause it to unfasten its talons. Unfortunately, I know only too well that our emotions are stronger than our reason; the man or woman at whose poor heart jealousy is gnawing day and night is not amenable to reason, is not curable by arguments; all we can do is to sympathize with such a person and ask the Lord to pity him or her.

I have known a man who lived with his wife in free union, i.e., he was not married to her. He did not believe in marriage. Love was the only bond that should bind people together; as soon as love was no more the people should separate in a friendly, comradely manner. If the wife or the mistress wants another lover, she should be free to take one; she is a free human being and not her husband's chattel slave, etc., etc., etc., to the same effect. Thus the man talked. And he was sincere in his talk—or he thought he was. But one night on unexpectedly returning home he found another man; he promptly fired several shots at the man, which fortunately for both did not prove fatal, and then he beat and choked his wife—who wasn't even his wife legally—within an inch of her life. *And then he married her* and gave up his free love talk. And I know of any number of men who could philosophize for hours about the disgrace and humiliation of being jealous, but who, as soon as there was a justifiable cause for jealousy, became as unreasonable as a child and as jealous as any unlettered Sicilian woman ever was.

So you see, I am not deluding myself with extravagant hopes. But, nevertheless, this argumentation, this talk, is not entirely useless. A beginning must be made. This essay may not perhaps help—except for the suggestions that will be made towards the end—those who are already victims of the demon of jealousy, but it may help some people to keep out of his clutches (or should I say: her clutches? I really don't know whether the demon of jealousy is a male or a female.)

Feelings are stronger than reason; but that does not mean that feelings cannot be influenced by reason; they decidedly can be and are so influenced, and their *manifestations* are modified by this influence; and the more cultured, the more educated a person is (I trust you will know that I use these terms in their true and not their vulgar, misused meaning), the more will his feelings, or at least actions, be influenced by his reason. I am particularly a believer in the effect on our feelings and actions of public opinion, of ideas universally or generally entertained.

Let me give one example which is pertinent to the subject. In former days it was universally held, and in many places it is still held, that when a wife sinned she committed the most unpardonable crime that a human being could be guilty of and that she thereby *dishonored* her husband. And the only right thing for him to do was to shoot the rival and cast out the wife; or at least to cast her out. This was a *conditio sine qua non*. To take her back to his home was a disgrace, a sign of unpardonable weakness, of degeneracy. Our ideas on the subject have changed a bit. A husband is no longer considered any more dishonored—in some strata of society at least—because his wife sinned than a wife is considered dishonored because her husband sinned; and adultery in the wife is now, by most rational people, considered only different in degree, but not in kind, from adultery in the husband. These humane ideas have gained vogue only within a comparatively very recent period; but their effect has already manifested itself in a great number of instances. Forgiving the erring wife is becoming quite common. A number of cases have reached the newspapers. Recently a wife was implicated in a nasty scrape; her sin was not only unquestionable, but notorious; it was public property. And nevertheless the husband stood by her and took her back into his home and arms. And the number of such cases which do not reach the newspapers is very, very much larger than the public has any conception of, larger than it would be safe to estimate. And in a large percentage of these cases the husband begins to treat his wife with more love, more consideration, and the tie between them becomes more firm, more permanent.

CHAPTER LII

REMEDIES FOR JEALOUSY

Prevention and Cure—Prophylaxis of Jealousy—Fitting Remedy to Circumstances—The Neglectful and Flirtatious Husband—No Question of Love—Advice to the wife of the Flirtatious Man—An Efficient Though Vulgar Remedy—Jealousy Must Be Experienced to Be Understood—Necessity for Freedom of Association—Lines of Conduct for the Wife—Contempt for a Certain Type of Wife and Husband—The Abandoned Lover—The Effects of Unrequited Love—Sublimated Sexual Desire—Replacing Unrequited Love—The Attitude of Goethe—Simultaneous Loves Possible—Successive Loves Possible—Eternal Loves—When Sex Relationships May Be Beneficial—Purchasable Sex Relations and Their Value—The Broken Engagement—The Terrible Effects on the Young Man—The Young Streetwalker—Sex Relations with Fiancé—Inundating Sense of Shame—Collapse—Attempts at Suicide—An Active Sex Life—The Results—The Prevention of Jealousy.

We are all agreed that prevention is more important than cure. But when a patient comes with a fully developed disease it is futile to speak to him of prevention. It is too late to sermonize. What he wants and what he needs is a cure, if such can be had. What has preceded has reference chiefly to the prophylaxis of jealousy, to the prevention of the development of this disease in the future.

The question is: Is there a *remedy* for this malady? Is there a *cure* for this horrible disease of jealousy?

The conditions are extremely complex, and the remedy must be fitted to the circumstances. Let us assume that the husband neglects his wife and causes her to be jealous, not because he is in love with another woman, but because he is flirtatious, light-headed, feather-brained and inconsiderate. Such cases are in the great majority. Many husbands who like or love their wives and who believe themselves secure in their love think it is quite proper for them to hunt for new conquests and to carry on petty love affairs with as many girls or women as they comfortably can. There is no question here about love—it is just flirtation or sexual relations. When this is the case the wife should have a frank and firm talk with her husband;

she should tell him that she does not like his behavior and that it makes her unhappy. In many instances this alone will suffice to effect a change in the husband's conduct. Where this does not suffice, where the husband is too egotistic and does not want to give up his little pleasures, then it is left for the wife to adopt the old and rather vulgar remedy. It is old and, as said, rather vulgar, but it has the merit of efficiency: it very often works. Let the wife adopt similar tactics, let her also flirt, let her go out and come back at uncertain hours, let her keep the husband guessing as to where and with whom she is. And nine times out of ten this, under the circumstances, fully justifiable conduct on the part of the wife will effect a quick and radical change in the conduct of the husband. He will be only too glad to cry quits. Some people are utterly devoid of imagination. They lack the ability of putting themselves in another person's place. Jealousy particularly is not a feeling which any one can understand without having experienced it, unless he is endowed with the imagination of a great poet. And as few husbands have a great poetic imagination, it is only after they have felt the claws of the monster tearing at their own hearts that they can understand their wives' feelings, and are willing to act so as to save them—and themselves, of course—the cruel tortures. Many wives and many husbands have talked to me and written to me on the subject, and, as stated before, in nine times out of ten the remedy worked.

But how about the tenth case? How about the cases where the husband is unable or unwilling to give up his outside flirtations and relations? We, advanced sexologists, know that not all men, no more than all women, are made in the same mould, and what is possible or even easy for nine men may be very difficult or absolutely impossible for the tenth. We know that there are some men to whom an ironclad monogamic relation is an absolute impossibility. The stimulation of other women—either the purely mental, spiritual stimulation or the stimulation of physical relations—is to them like breath in the nostrils. In fact, there are some men whose very possibility of loving their wives depends upon this freedom of association with other women. They can be extremely kind to and love their wives tenderly, if they can at the same time associate—spiritually or physically—with other women. If they are entirely cut off from any association with any other woman they begin to feel irritable, bored, may become ill, and their feeling towards their wives may become one of resentment, ill-will, or even one of hatred.

This is not the place to talk of the wickedness of such men—thus they are made and with this fact we have to deal.

What is the wife of such a man to do? Two lines of conduct are open to her—two avenues of exit. The line of conduct will depend upon her temper and upon her ideas of sex morality. But she ought to select the line of conduct which will cause the least pain, the least unhappiness. If she is a woman of a proud, independent temper, particularly if she belongs to the militant type, she will leave her husband in a huff, regardless of consequences. But if she is a woman of the gentler, more pliable, more supple (and I may also say more subtle) type, and if she really loves her husband, she will overlook his little foibles, peccadilloes and transgressions—and she may live quite happily. And the time will come when the husband himself will give up his peccadilloes and transgressions and will cleave powerfully to his wife, will be bound to her by bonds never to be torn asunder. *I know of several such cases.*

And I will take this opportunity to say that I have the deepest contempt for the wife who, on finding out that her husband had committed a transgression or that he has a love affair, leaves him in a huff, or makes a public scandal, or sues for divorce. Such a wife *never* loved her husband, and he is well rid of her. And what I said about the wife applies with *almost* equal force to the husband.

The Abandoned Lover. But what shall the abandoned lover do? Let us take the case of A and B, and let A stand for any man and B for any woman; or, *vice versa*, let A be the woman and B the man, for in jealousy and love what applies to one sex is applicable with practically the same force to the opposite sex. Suppose A is intensely jealous of and deeply, passionately in love with B; but B is utterly indifferent and does not care what A may feel or do. A and B may be married or not; this does not alter the case materially. Suppose B, if unmarried to A, goes off and marries another man, or, if married to A, goes off and leaves him; or suppose B does not love anybody else, but just remains indifferent to A's advances or repels him because she cannot reciprocate his love. Unrequited love alone can cause almost as fierce tortures as the most intense jealousy. And A suffers tortures. What shall he do? What shall he do to save himself—to save his health, his mind, his life? For he is unable to eat, unable to sleep, unable to work, and he feels that he is going to pieces. He has lost his position and is in danger of losing his reason. What shall he do to escape insanity or a suicide's grave? There is but one remedy. Let him use all his energies to find a *substitute*. I mean a living substitute. Mere sexual desire may be sublimated, to a certain extent, into other channels, may be replaced by work, study, a hobby or some engrossing interest. A great unrequited love, with the element of jealousy present or absent, cannot be replaced by anything else except by another love. And where as great a love is impossible let it be a minor love or a series of minor loves. When Goethe, one of the world's great lovers, was unable to walk in the broad avenue of a great love he would walk in the by-paths of a number of little loves. The common talk about a person being unable to love more than once in his or her life is silly nonsense. A man or a woman is able to love, and love very deeply, a number of times; and love simultaneously or successively. It is often a mere matter of opportunity. I know that there *are* loves that are eternal; that there are loves for which no substitute can be found. But these supreme, divine loves are so rare that among ordinary mortals they may be left out of account. They are the portion of supermen and superwomen. Ordinarily a substitute may be found. The substitute love may never reach the intensity of the original love, it may never give full or even half-full satisfaction; but it will help to dull the sharp cutting edge, it will act as a partial hemostatic to the bleeding heart, it will soothe and anesthetize the wound even if it cannot completely heal it. And this is a valuable aid while the sufferer is coming to himself or herself, while the gathered fragments of a broken life are being cemented and while the cement is hardening. Yes, the man or woman who is in inferno on account of an unreciprocated or a betrayed love should lose no time in searching for a substitute love. I do not believe in people losing their health and their minds on account of suffering which does nobody any good.

But I will go still further. Where a substitute love—great or minor— cannot be found, then mere sex relations may help to diminish the suffering, to quiet the turbulent heart, to relieve the aching brain. As everything connected with sex, so our ideas about illicit sex relations that are not connected with love, are honeycombed with hypocrisy and false to the core. While purchasable, loveless sex relations can, of course, not be compared to love relations, still under our present social, economic and moral code they are the only relations that thousands of men and women can enjoy, and they are better than none; and in quite a considerable percentage of cases an element of romance and greater or lesser permanency do become attached to them, and they act as a more or less satisfactory substitute for genuine love relations.

I am not spinning theoretical gossamer webs. I am speaking from experience—the experience of patients and confiding friends. I could relate many interesting cases. And I may, in a more appropriate volume. Here one or two will have to suffice.

He was twenty-six years old and a senior student in the College of Physicians and Surgeons, Columbia University, New York. He had been in love with and had considered himself engaged for four or five years to a young lady two years his junior. She was, of course, the most wonderful young lady in the world, the whole world; in fact, there was not another one to compare her to. She was unique; she stood all alone. But for a year or so she was getting rather cool towards him; which fanned his flame all the more. And suddenly he received a note asking him not to call any more, nor to try to communicate in any other way. He did write, but his letters were returned unopened. And soon after he read of her engagement to a prominent young banker. He nearly went insane, and this is used not in any figurative sense. His insomnia was *complete,* and resisted all treatment. When his pulse became very rapid and his eyes acquired the wild look that they do after many sleepless nights an attempt was made to administer hypnotics, but they had practically no effect. Chloral, veronal, etc., only made him "dopy," irritable and depressed, but did not give him one hour of sound sleep. His appetite was gone, now and then his limbs would twitch, and he would sit and stare into space for hours at a time. To study or attend the clinics was out of the question, and he did not even attempt to take the final examinations. The parents felt distressed, but were unable to do anything for him. The least attempt at interference on their part, any attempt to console him, to induce him to pull himself together, made him more irritable, more morose; so that they finally left him alone. He was practically a total abstainer, but one evening he went out and came home drunk; and after that he drank frequently and heavily. His parents could do nothing with him. One evening on Broadway he was accosted by a young street-walker. She had a pleasant, sympathetic face, and he went with her. *That was his first sex experience.* Up to that time he was chaste. He met her again the following evening. Gradually a sort of friendship grew up between them. She found out the cause of his grief, and with maternal solicitude she tried everything in her power to console him, and he began to look forward to the nightly meeting with her. His grief became gradually less acute, he gave up drinking, which he disliked, and which he had taken up only to deaden his pain; he began to pull himself together, and in six or eight months he took over his last year in Columbia and was properly graduated. He kept up the friendship with the girl for over two years, when she died of pneumonia. He did not love her, but he liked to be with her, as her presence gave him physical and mental comfort. It is possible that she loved him genuinely, but there was never any sentimental talk between them, and there was never any question between them of the permanency of the relationship. They both knew that it was temporary. But he is absolutely certain that but for one of the representatives of the class that is despised, driven about and persecuted by brutal policemen and ignorant judges, he would have become a bum, or, most likely, he would have committed suicide— at the point of which he was several times; only pity for his mother and sisters restrained him.

And here is another case. A girl about twenty-eight years of age fell in love with a man four or five years her senior. The love seemed to be reciprocated, and they soon became engaged to be married. He asked that the engagement, on account of certain business reasons, be kept secret. She did not know the man well; she had met him at several entertainments and church affairs and he seemed very nice. He always found some excuses for delaying the marriage, and after they had been engaged about a year he began to insist on sex relations. Though of a refined and noble character, she was of a passionate nature and she did not offer much resistance. Many girls who would under no circumstance indulge in illicit relations, considering it a great sin, have no compunctions about having relations with their fiancés. They lived together for about a year. They were together almost daily, except now and then, when he would go away for a week or two on business. Once he went away— and never came back. He wrote to her that their relations were at an end; that he was a married man and a father of children; he had hoped he might get a divorce, but that now he had changed his mind and that she must forget him, etc. Everything was black before her. It cost her a supreme effort not to faint, and she was supported in this effort by the fact that when the letter came she was in the presence of friends; a terrible, overpowering, all-inundating sense of shame gave her the strength not to betray her condition and her story before the world at large. But as soon as she was alone she collapsed completely. There was the most absolute insomnia imaginable, complete anorexia, but the most distressing features were frequent fainting spells, severe palpitation of the heart and tremors. She had no love for the man—so she said. Her love had turned to hatred and contempt—but the jealousy was all-consuming. Like a fire it was burning in her, searing her brain and her soul day and night.

She felt that she was not strong enough to stand this physical and mental torture, and so she decided to commit suicide. As the means she selected gas. Fortunately, the smell became perceptible before the injury was irreparable. She was saved. But she felt that she could not stand the torture very long—and more than anything was she afraid that her mind would give way. She had a special horror of insanity. And so she decided to make another attempt This time with bichloride. Again she was saved. A friend of hers then got an inkling of the events that were transpiring, and she introduced her to some gentlemen friends. They were nice people and more or less radical on the sex question. In order to drown her pain she began to go out very frequently with that crowd, and to her surprise and delight she found that she soon began to think less and less about her contemptible seducer, and, what was more important to her, she was soon able to sleep. For about six months she led an extremely active, almost promiscuous sex life. But then she gave it up, as she felt herself normal and no longer in need of it. She is now happily married.

I am through with this rather lengthy essay on one of the most painful manifestations of human emotional life. I repeat that I am aware that feelings are often stronger than reason; but saying this does not mean asserting that feelings cannot be modified and held in check by reason. And I feel confident that a careful, open-minded reading of these pages and an acceptance of the ideas therein promulgated would aid in *preventing* a good deal of the misery of jealousy and in curing a certain proportion of it after it has found lodgment in the hearts of unhappy men and women.

There are one or two more points that might be touched upon, but with the freedom of press in reference to sex matters as it exists in this country to-day, I have said all that I could say.

CHAPTER LIII

CONCLUDING WORDS

It is my sincere belief—and I cherish the belief in spite of this horrible, wretched war which seems to be shattering the very foundations of everything that we hold dear, destroying all the humane and moral achievements that have been laboriously built up in the course of many centuries—that the time will come when the world will be practically free from pain and suffering. Almost all disease will be conquered, accidents will be rare, the fear of starvation or poverty or unemployment will no longer haunt men and women, every infant born will be well-born and welcome, and the numerous anxieties and ambitions that now disturb the lives of so many of the earth's inhabitants will no longer plague us. They will be the dead memories of a dead and forgotten past.

Yes, I believe that the time will come when the world will be practically free from pain and suffering. But there is one exception. I do not believe that we will ever be able entirely to eliminate the *tragedies of the heart*. For our physical ills, which will be few in number, there will be a socialized medical profession; everywhere there will be free hospitals and convalescent homes. The unemployment problem will be dealt with by the State, and dealt with so that there will be no unemployment problem. There will be work for everybody and everybody will do the work which he finds most congenial. But the State, I fear, will be able to do nothing in affairs of the heart. When John loves Mary with every fiber of his soul, and Mary remains completely indifferent, then no State physician and no Government official will be able to offer any balm or consolation to poor John. And if Mary loves Robert, and Robert behaves so that he breaks Mary's heart, then no official glue will put it together and no convalescent home will make it whole.

Yes, I believe that love pangs and tragedies of the heart will cause mortal men and women suffering even under the most perfect social regime. But I also believe that these pangs will be less acute, that the suffering will be less cruel than it is now.

Proper ideas about love, freer intercourse between the sexes, a normal and regular sex life, a saner attitude towards many things which are now unjustly considered shameful or criminal will, to a large degree, prevent the heart tragedies and facilitate their cure where they cannot be prevented.

And it is the duty of everybody who loves mankind to study the various phases of human sexuality and help to spread sane and humane ideas on the subject of Sex and Love.

The author trusts that Woman: Her Sex and Love Life will help, in some slight degree, in spreading healthy, sane and honest ideas about sex among the men and women of America.

OTHER TITLES

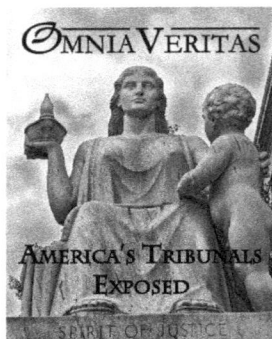

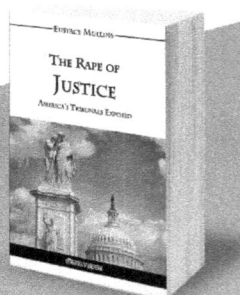

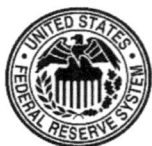

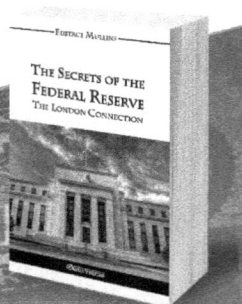

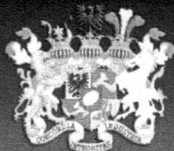

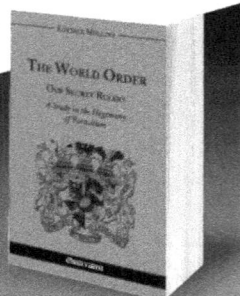

OMNIA VERITAS. Omnia Veritas Ltd presents:

FREDERICK SODDY

THE ROLE OF MONEY

FREDERICK SODDY

THE ROLE OF MONEY

WHAT IT SHOULD BE CONTRASTED
WITH WHAT IT HAS BECOME

This book attempts to clear up the mystery of money in its social aspect

This, surely, is what the public really wants to know about money

OMNIA VERITAS. Omnia Veritas Ltd presents:

FREDERICK SODDY

WEALTH, VIRTUAL WEALTH AND DEBT

FREDERICK SODDY

WEALTH, VIRTUAL WEALTH AND DEBT

THE SOLUTION OF THE ECONOMIC PARADOX

The most powerful tyranny and the most universal conspiracy against the economic freedom of individuals and the autonomy of nations the world has yet known.

THE SOLUTION OF THE ECONOMIC PARADOX

The public are most carefully shielded from any real knowledge...

OMNIA VERITAS. Omnia Veritas Ltd presents:

Confessions of a BRITISH SPY

It is no wonder that Wahhabis are now the backbone of terrorism, authorising, financing and planning the shedding of the blood of Muslims and other innocents.

British enmity against Islam

Confessions of a BRITISH SPY

This document reveals the true context of the Wahhabi movement

www.ingramcontent.com/pod-product-compliance
Lightning Source LLC
Chambersburg PA
CBHW061721270326
41928CB00011B/2073